for A.

Down Is
Up
for Aaron Eagle

A Mother's Spiritual Journey with
Down Syndrome

و

VICKI NOBLE

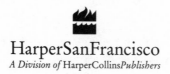

HarperSanFrancisco
A Division of HarperCollins*Publishers*

FIRST EDITION

Library of Congress Cataloging-in-Publication Data
Noble, Vicki.
    Down is up for Aaron Eagle : a mother's spiritual journey with
Down syndrome / Vicki Noble. — 1st ed.
        p.   cm.
    Includes bibliographical references.
    ISBN 0-06-250737-0 (pbk.)
    1. Noble, Aaron Eagle, 1985– . 2. Down's syndrome — Patients —
Biography. 3. Down's syndrome — Patients — Family relationships.
4. Down's syndrome — Religious aspects — New Age movement.
I. Title.
RJ506.D68N635 1993
362. 1'96858842'0092 — dc20
    [B]   92–56118
                                                           CIP

93 94 95 96 97 ❖ HAD 10 9 8 7 6 5 4 3 2 1

This edition is printed on acid-free paper that meets the American National Standards Institute Z39.48 Standard.

Song to Aaron Eagle*

Aaron is his Mama's boy
Aaron is his Daddy's joy
Aaron is our special boy
Aaron Eagle boy.

I love Aaron Eagle
He's my special boy
I love Aaron Eagle
He fills my heart with joy.

Night-night, Aaron Eagle
Night-night, little boy of mine
Night-night, Aaron Eagle
Night-night, little one.

*I have sung this song to Aaron Eagle for so long that he now requests it at bedtime along with the accompanying back rub before he sleeps.

Contents

Acknowledgments

ॐ

Obviously, this book is dedicated to Aaron Eagle, the shaman boy.

In the text itself, I've basically named everyone whom I need to thank for helping in Aaron's daily life—his daddy, our friends and extended family, all those who love and look after him and who have intervened in helping ways in our life with him.

I want to acknowledge those people who particularly helped me with the book itself. I am indebted to Khara Whitney-Marsh, Elinor Gadon, Karen Vogel, Amy Opalk, Gloria Nailor, and Jennifer Berezan for careful, critical readings of the manuscript at various stages of writing and rewriting. Jennifer, especially, hung in there with it until the very last days, giving it more than one thorough going-over and helping me bring it satisfactorily to completion. Khara and Jennifer also each spent time in libraries, finding the odd detail I needed to know about Down syndrome, eagles, or what have you. Thank you, everybody.

Vicki Noble
April 25, 1993

Introduction

༈

THIS MORNING WAS A RED LETTER DAY AT OUR house; Aaron Eagle had an intellectual breakthrough. After breakfast, he looked at the bag lunch sitting on the counter and asked, "Aaron, school lunch—cookie, chips?" I laughed and told him no, there were no cookies or chips in his lunch today. I opened the lunch, showing him the banana, yogurt, and juice I had packed for him.

"School lunch," he repeated patiently, "cookie? Chips?" He seemed to be watching intently for my response. Then nodding with more self-assurance, he demanded, "Chips!"

I added a small bag of organic blue corn chips to his lunch. He nodded again, pleased with himself and life, and went off to school. In order to accomplish that simple task, he had to anticipate the future (his lunch, hours from now) and remember the past (yesterday's apparently inferior lunch lacking a cookie or chips) and initiate an action in regard to this conceptual understanding (getting me to change the lunch). For a child with Down syndrome, that's a minor miracle.

I'd like to share with you what it's like living with Aaron Eagle, a modern boy with the chromosomal abnormality known as Down syndrome who rarely thinks of the past or anticipates the future. I was lucky enough in my midlife passage to become the mother of this special boy who shows me every day how to "be here now." I often ponder the fact that spiritual teachers urge us to focus on the moment and to find meaning in the most mundane events. Eating, elimination, breathing—these are the raw stuff of spiritual practice. Having been Aaron Eagle's mom for eight years now, I have learned much by watching him make his humble way in the world.

I'd like to ask all the "normal" people who read this book to consider the hypothesis that those whom we think of as "disabled" and "handicapped" might paradoxically be embodiments of divinity who have manifested to wake us up from our assumptions. Our modern Western culture doesn't recognize the role of what shamanistic cultures have called the trickster or sacred clown, or else special people like Aaron Eagle would surely be seen as such.

There are a hundred examples I could give. One memorable Sunday morning Aaron Eagle, his daddy Jonathan, and I were taking a leisurely walk along College Avenue in

Berkeley, California, on our way to have breakfast in a favorite restaurant. We passed a bus stop bench where an elderly African-American woman was sitting. She seemed lost in her own world, perhaps a bit sad or low, and Aaron, who was about two and a half years old at the time, responded to some need in her with his typically bright spirit. "Hi," he said as he made a detour and went over to shake her hand and give her five. Then he babbled in his own special language, gesturing and laughing. She was so touched, she began to weep. She looked around at us and said, "It's the hand a' God on him." She repeated this phrase over and over, tears streaming down her face in a moment of ecstasy, while Aaron smiled and said a casual, satisfied "bye-bye" to her.

It is indeed the hand of the Divine on this child, and apparently on others with Down syndrome. Every person with Down syndrome whom I have ever met seemed happier, friendlier, more congenial and kindhearted than the rest of us, and I've heard other people say this as well. For the last fifteen years, I have been on a spiritual journey intended to develop just such qualities in myself. All paths of the Eastern spiritual disciplines—Buddhism, Taoism, yoga—as well as progressive Christianity and Judaism, are theoretically focused on opening the heart and developing compassion for all beings. People with Down syndrome seem to have this gift naturally; they are born with it.

Those with Down syndrome belong to a special family. They have features that cause them to look alike, even when they also look like their biological families. They have a sort

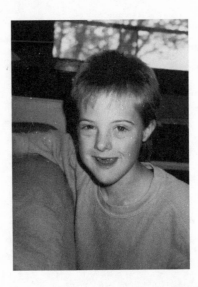

Aaron Eagle with
his two front
teeth missing,
age eight.
Photo by
Karen Vogel.

of tribal resemblance, as if they are all related. Aaron re-
cently saw the cover of a contemporary magazine, *Down
Syndrome Today,* featuring an article on twin boys with
Down syndrome. He pointed to the boys and said, "Aaron."

Technically, people with Down syndrome are not missing
anything. Rather they have one extra chromosome, which
gives them almond-shaped eyes and arched palates, and apparently causes them to be peculiarly open, happy, and giving. What they seem to lack is ego, and in Western culture
that is perceived as a horrendous loss. Yet I often envy
Aaron's uncluttered simplicity. He has very few preferences,
and the ones he has took a long time to develop. He likes
trucks, hats, trolls, and harmonicas. Over the years, he has
worked hard to learn to say "my" and "mine," and "this," not
"that." Yet a Buddhist might work an entire lifetime (or

more) on ridding the ego of its attachments and preferences, which are perceived as the root cause of suffering.

The New Age movement in the United States (and now around the world) has borrowed ideas from Eastern religion, such as the open heart and the bodhisattva of compassion. "New Age" people talk about opening the heart and being compassionate, when in real life we sometimes seem more concerned about ourselves and our own narrow world of personal drama, which we have mistakenly equated with "spiritual" development. When our concerns do not extend beyond the narcissistic world of our individual pain (how my parents hurt me, how the world doesn't receive me, how difficult my life is because I am the child of an alcoholic, etc.), then our goals are often reduced to getting more of what's out there (you create your own reality; you can have it all).

Yet the ultimate goal of all spiritual work is service, and the means of attaining the goal is practice. The Vietnamese Buddhist monk Thich Nhat Hanh has said, "One does not become enlightened. Enlightenment is the way."[1] One must practice serving, helping, giving, caring, reaching out without attachment or investment in outcome. This altruism is understandably difficult, and we lack sufficient role models for it, but experience has shown that it can be developed through practices that literally open the heart.

People with Down syndrome are gifted with this genuine way of being. Why then is it so difficult for us to recognize them as the bodhisattvas among us? A bodhisattva, in Tibetan Buddhism, is a person (or a deity) who, on be-coming free, rather than leaving the wheel of continuous rebirth chooses instead to reincarnate over and over again, helping to free others, until everyone is free. The bodhi-sattva path is a path of loving service and compassionate outreach. The archaic words used in the not-so-distant past to describe people with Down syndrome (retarded, simple-minded, mongoloids, imbeciles, idiots) have obscured their divinity, and this obscuring particularly blinds us to the ways they are perhaps more evolved than the rest of us. Our society spent decades putting them away in institu-tions, getting them out of our sight, when we might have been following their lead and learning how to behave from the example they set.

I worry about the way in which technology has devel-oped routine amniocentesis, so that any woman can know in advance that she carries a child with Down syndrome and make a supposedly informed choice about whether or not to carry her pregnancy to term. As a feminist activist, I have no conflicts about a woman's right to choose any form of birth control, and abortion when all else fails. But I'm worried about the seeming consensus that a woman would naturally not want to give birth to a child with "chromo-somal damage," in other words, a child like Aaron Eagle. I'm worried about the powerful unspoken agreement in this modern medical approach that wants to eliminate "de-fectives" from the population. Does the mother in this case actually have any intuitive say in the decision? Can she feel her own feelings and needs, in the face of so much pressure from authorities? A woman needs space to feel her child as that child actually is, rather than through the philosophical lens of an opinionated public.

I have been a healer for fifteen years. I have studied and practiced yoga, meditation, chanting, self-development, trance techniques, shamanic journeying, Tarot, astrology, and hands-on healing. I've looked at the research suggesting that Down syndrome may be caused by radiation from early childhood dental and medical X rays (of which I had many), and the higher incidence of Down syndrome, as well as other birth defects, at places where nuclear reactors have leaked or uranium tailings are found. Dr. Robert Mendelsohn stated in 1979 that mothers who have given birth to children with Down syndrome have had seven times the dental and medical X rays of mothers of comparable age who have given birth to normal children.[2] Radiation is known to cause species mutations, because of its seemingly random splitting of cells. Unfortunately, we have no comparative records of the incidence of Down syndrome from earlier times, before there was so much radiation used so casually.

What if people with Down syndrome are a mutation and part of their inherent makeup is that their hearts are spiritually wide open? What would stop us then from seeing them as living embodiments of evolution, instead of seeing them as defective? Wouldn't we then care for them, and study and learn from them? This is not to deny that they are developmentally delayed. Aaron Eagle still can't reliably use the toilet at the age of eight, and his talking is somewhat hit-and-miss. But I know it's not easy to admit that our Western scientific, technological, linear, hyper-rational, and frenetic approach to life might not be the best one, and that these "slower" people have something we ourselves might need.

I would even go so far as to suggest that people with Down syndrome may very well represent a way in which the human species is groping toward a new form. They aren't perfect, but they are certainly not a failed experiment! Their very simplicity is the piece we are missing in our twentieth-century puzzle. Look at Thich Nhat Hanh, whose focused appreciation while eating a piece of fruit is the basis of his spiritual teaching, or the Nobel Prize–winning Dalai Lama, who emphasizes that he is a simple peasant man yet carries the highest spiritual and secular authority for Tibetans in and outside Tibet. Aaron often seems as much like a Zen monk as practicing Zen monks are!

I don't mean to make light of Aaron's disability or to deny that at times I wish he were able to relate on a more sophisticated level. I am simply suggesting that who he is, in and of itself, has something to offer the rest of us. His way of being is a cogent fragment of what we are missing in our modern society, and he demonstrates unequivocally what it would take for us to bring our world back into balance. Of course, when Aaron makes a leap to a more complex level of intellectual understanding, as he did this morning in relation to his lunch, I am always thrilled. I am happy that such leaps are possible, and that his future is unknown. It used to be that no one expected anything of children with Down syndrome, and now no one knows what each child might be capable of learning and doing.

This book is a mother's attempt to communicate the wonder and beauty of a child with Down syndrome. I am so proud of Aaron Eagle! He has to work so much harder than the rest of us to do the simplest things, and as a result his gains are more profound than ours. We take so much of life for granted, forgetting to be appreciative of the little pleasures or truly grateful for the big achievements. The look on Aaron's face when he accomplishes something ordinary for the first time is a spiritual doorway for the most jaded among us. He has to focus on putting one foot in front of the other just to climb the stairs every day, yet he rarely complains or whines about his difficulties.

I want the world for Aaron. I want a world in which children are loved and cared for, each of them wanted from the first moment, all of them given what they need. I want children to be seen as a top priority in our society's responsibility toward its people, with their protection guaranteed and their safety assured. I want peace on earth and food for everyone, an end to war and violence, and a departure from greed and profit as the central motivating forces behind everything. I can bear the breakdown that's occurring in modern civilization if it means that we are forced to learn again the simple things like sharing and community. A person like Aaron

Eagle "pops us out of our dramas," as John McGowan (an adult person with Down syndrome) stated it, and helps us "to get our love flows going."[3]

My book is a story of Aaron's life and the people who love him, as well as an effort to advocate for him and others like him. I want to break down the stereotypes about "retarded" people and about children in general. My point of view is that of a healer, as well as a mother, and my approach to the world is a somewhat radical one. I don't expect that everyone will agree with me, but I think everyone can learn something from Aaron Eagle and the other people with Down syndrome among us today. Aaron Eagle's particular context includes an alternative approach to diet, medicine, and religion that I believe is supporting him develop his functioning to as high a level as possible.

"Our children are all that we need, if we'd just get out of their way," sings our family friend Jennifer Berezan.[4] Our basic approach to Aaron Eagle has been to watch and wait, letting him show us the direction in which he would like to go. We try to intuit what he needs, rather than forcing him down a certain preselected track. We respond to what he asks for and support and encourage his initiative in any direction. Because he has responded so strongly to music, we continually present him with musical opportunities; because he likes to play ball, we have provided a basketball coach and a golf teacher. Whenever he reaches out toward something, we try our best to create a space wherein he can make contact with that thing and achieve it. Nothing seems out of the question, and other than becoming toilet trained and talking clearly, nothing seems mandatory either.

The chapters in this book are in a kind of loose chronological order, but I ask that you keep in mind that Aaron Eagle is only eight years old, so I cannot possibly write the story of his life. He is like a flower just beginning to blossom, and these chapters are only my impressionistic glimpses into his expression of himself as I see it now. His daddy and I think Aaron Eagle is a healer—a "wounded healer," or shaman, to be exact—and that, like all healers everywhere, he is "called" to do a certain work. He has had a transformative impact on our lives, and on those of the other people close to him, and he seems to have the ability to reach outside our extended family, affecting and transforming the lives of total strangers as well.

His love of theater and a microphone, his ease in being at the center of groups of any size, and his enthusiastic urge to perform for any audience make us think he will someday be a performer in his own right, and that the healing he is born to do will be done through that channel. But first the basics: he will have to learn to carry a tune, speak in a language we can all recognize, and go to the bathroom in a toilet without being reminded! In a way, Aaron embodies the extremes that are the potential in human nature, modeling both our deficits and our best efforts. Although I cannot possibly provide an unbiased report on him, I hope to describe a range of behaviors and idiosyncratic characteristics that express his soul and personality.

I know without a doubt that the parents of other children with Down syndrome will recognize their own child in Aaron, and I can't help but hope that "normal" people will see themselves in him as well. Since Aaron's birth, I have had several dreams in which there is a little girl, who is actually me, who is handicapped and suffering many of the pains and struggles that afflict Aaron Eagle. I think this is the deepest truth about disabilities and probably explains an irrational fear of the people who embody them. Within each one of us is a damaged child with hidden wounds that are the source of unrelieved pain and suffering. The pain from these wounds could be the source of healing if it were brought to the surface and released. Stuck inside us, it festers and causes us to build defenses and create strategies that keep us from the intimacy and love we crave. Surely it is this armoring that allows conflict to grow into wars — and allows domestic violence to exist at all. I believe that in a magical and nonrational way, being around Aaron Eagle, who is visibly wounded but does not feel sorry for himself, we are mirrored back to ourselves in wholeness and completion.

If our hearts can open to "disabled" people so that we can actually experience them as themselves, rather than experiencing only our fear of them, we can find the innate compassion in ourselves to embrace all of what is in each one of us. For not only is Aaron's wound right there for all to see, but his profound courage and determination are a sight for sore eyes, as well. When I say, as I will in this book, that Aaron Eagle is my teacher, I am not waxing lyrical in a deluded, Pollyanna-type state of denial. I am not feeling sorry for him or trying to compensate by thinking up nice things to say about him. I am simply telling the truth as I can best express it. In some way, Aaron came from the Mystery, and he brings some of it with him into my life and the lives of others. It is this mysterious gift of his that made me want to write this book.

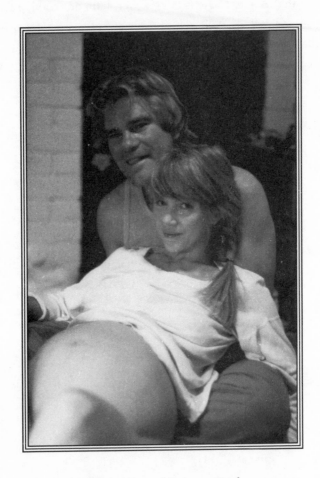

Vicki in labor with Aaron Eagle;
supporting is Jonathan Tenney, Aaron's father.
Photo by Brooke Ziegler.

Chapter One

A Magical Child
Is Born

꒰

ONCE UPON A TIME, THERE WAS A MODERN MAN AND A modern woman, and they met and fell in love. Naturally, they decided to get married and have a baby. Never mind that they were in their middle age, and never mind that they already had two babies each who were almost grown up by now. Dreams instilled in early childhood die hard. Both the woman and the man were divorced from the first spouse, and they longed to fulfill the childhood dream of Cinderella and the prince living happily ever after. When our dreams fail to come true the first time, we often try again. So it was with the future parents of little Aaron Eagle, the shaman boy.

I want to tell you the story of Aaron Eagle, but I can't tell you about him without first returning to his origins. He was invented as part of a myth that his father and I had decided to live out. This mythic background seems crucial for an understanding of who we think he is and how much he means to us.

Jonathan and I met and became friends in 1982. For a year, we nourished our relationship without allowing it to become "romantic." Finally, after long deliberation, we took the plunge. I left the man I lived with and joined with the wild Dionysian lover I saw in Jonathan. Within three months of becoming lovers, we were married and attempting to get me pregnant. We already knew the name of the child we wanted to bring into this world: Aaron Eagle. If the child was a girl, her last name would be Noble-Tenney; a boy would carry his father's name first and be Tenney-Noble. We even debated about the spelling of the first name, should the child be a girl, and settled on Aaryn Eagle.

Our marriage had been divinely ordained. Two weeks from our first night together, I had the following dream:

I am hiking along with my partner, and suddenly, sitting very still just ahead of us, is a bald eagle. I stop and look and wait to see what will happen. I am very excited, having always wanted to see such a wonderful bird.

Somehow, the next thing I know, the eagle is taking me with him to be his partner. He wants to make me — or he recognizes me as — one of the Light Beings, and he takes me as his mate. I leave my partner reluctantly, but unhesitatingly, since this higher calling pulls me without reservation. There is to be a marriage. Even while I am in a state of wonder that such a thing is possible, I surrender to it. I am to become an eagle myself now in the transformation process of union with him.

Eagles pair-bond for life, sometimes mating for fifty years. Ignoring the signs of the times, such as the high divorce rate in California and the fact that most children do not live in families that include both their biological parents, Jonathan and I pushed ahead toward manifestation of the dream. We were married on Friday, May 27th, in Mérida, the beautiful capital of Yucatán. The man who officiated at the courthouse wedding did so with little fanfare, as he spoke only Spanish and we knew only a few phrases ourselves. Imagine our disbelief and wonder when he signed his name to our marriage certificate: Señor Aguilar, Mr. Eagle. When we returned home that summer to Santa Cruz, California, we invited a hundred guests to our home in the country to witness and celebrate our union. At this second wedding celebration, a photographer took pictures of the ceremony, and in one of the photos—when I am putting Jonathan's ring on his finger—in the background is a distinct figure of a bald eagle, created from nothing more than the play of light on the leaves of the tree under which we stood to say our vows.

The first time I got pregnant we were both still very sick from our stay in Mexico, which had ended badly. We had spent a week in Mexico City, sick as dogs, stuck in our hotel room and waiting for money that, due to some mix-up with the telex machines, never arrived from the States. On Summer Solstice, June 21st, Jonathan's mother was finally

17

able to get us plane tickets home from her side, and we staggered to the airport, slept on the floor overnight, and caught an early flight to Phoenix, where we had left our car. It took a year to fully recover from the dysentery or whatever it was we had contracted our first night in Mexico City. After five weeks of being fairly careful about what we ate in Mexico, we had thrown caution to the winds and, in a moment of spontaneity, bought sweet corn from a vendor in the *zocalo* (the town square). I can still conjure up the smell of the water the man was pouring over the steaming corn to keep it hot.

So the first pregnancy did not come to much. Less than two months into it, I miscarried on Winter Solstice, exactly six months after leaving Mexico. Jonathan and I grieved that my body had not been healthier and more able to carry the child we both wanted. I visited a Chinese acupuncturist, who helped me regain my strength so that we could consider trying again. By the spring, we had just about decided to give up the idea of having our own child together. It seemed to go against the grain a bit, given our ages and that we each had already raised a first family. I thought it wouldn't be long before we would be turned into grandparents by one of our four daughters.

One night I awoke in the middle of the night with a strong urge to move away from California to "somewhere hot and dry." (In those days, it rained here all winter!) I was worried about earthquakes, and I was attracted to withdrawing into a semi-seclusion for a while. We threw the *I Ching* and got "the Creative," the number-one hexagram, without any changes. What that advice told us was that we were obliged to simply act without questioning our decision. We decided right then, at four in the morning, that we would pack up and move to the Southwest. I fantasized that we would eventually organize a healing center there that people would come to from all over the country, but that was never more than a thoughtform. Sometime in the ensuing months, we "doused" on a map of the Southwest to find our location. With a crystal hanging from a chain and a needle that we stuck into the dots representing towns on the map, we found our future dwelling place: Cornville, Arizona, perfect for a corn-fed Iowa girl like me and twenty miles south of the famous Sedona, with its legendary "vortex" energies.

On the day before we left for Arizona, when we got the moving truck and brought it home, I noticed I was nauseous as I was brushing my teeth. With a shock, I realized I was pregnant! I couldn't figure out when it had happened, but in that moment, everything slipped into place. No wonder we were moving to the country, we were going to have a baby! We happily headed off to begin our new life, arriving at our destination on August 1st (the Lammas holiday on the sacred calendar), with the temperature in Cornville at 110 degrees in the shade. Our new home was idyllic—a small, hand-built adobe house with a courtyard and willow trees all around. Beautiful Oak Creek flowed through our backyard, with red rock cliffs and blue herons making it a paradise. (Jonathan had driven out ahead and found this place in less than twenty-four hours. Once again we felt that what happened to us had been divinely ordained.) We settled in, planting a garden, and had fresh greens for my dinner in a matter of weeks.

Every day I walked the road that led to the cliffs above the river. Sometimes Jonathan and I crossed the river, and he jogged while I took a more leisurely walk. During these times, I was at peace in a way I had never been before. I felt a kinship with the land and with the tribal people who had lived on that land for millennia. I would walk across the desert thinking that I was a pregnant woman walking through the desert the way pregnant women had done since the beginning of human evolution. One day while I was walking above the creek, I heard a rattling sound that wasn't familiar. Lost in reverie, I continued to walk until the sound happened again, and the rattlesnake penetrated my consciousness. I stopped in my tracks, and there she was—an enormous diamondback rattler, four or five feet long, either pregnant or with a rather large dinner in her belly. She was sluggishly making her way along the side of the road, and we eyed each other with interest. When I would approach too close, she would rear up and rattle gently; when I stayed my distance, she simply watched me. I was completely delighted and sang to her: "Open mine eyes that I may see, glimpses of truth Thou hast for me; open mine eyes, illumine me, Spirit divine."[1] The rattlesnake was a special animal to me, and I had longed to meet one in just this way. I felt utterly blessed by the encounter.

At some point early in my pregnancy, I began to spot again, just as I had done with my miscarriage one year earlier. I went to a natural healer I had heard about, who was very helpful and supportive, and then I came home and told Jonathan I was losing the baby. We held each other and cried for two hours, then went to bed, having entirely surrendered to our fate. I had lost perhaps a tablespoonful of blood at that point. In the morning, there was no more blood, and I seemed to be still perfectly pregnant. It was only at that point that it began to really hit home that we might carry this baby to term and be parents together, as we had hoped. What a relief, to begin to feel safely pregnant!

In the healer's office, I had mentioned that I was looking for a midwife. He knew just the person, and after our almost-miscarriage, I called her. She lived an hour north of us in Flagstaff, in a beautiful rural setting, where we met with her the first time. An unlicensed midwife, she was afraid her status might be a liability for us and encouraged us to shop around. I laughed and said she was just what we were looking for! "What's that?" she asked. "Absolutely no medical intervention," I answered, and we bonded immediately.

Later she visited me in my home, with the woman who was her labor partner and would assist at our birth. My two midwives came regularly to visit me. It was lovely interacting with these two country women, with all their earthy wisdom that came from all the natural births they had attended over the years. They would come to our house by the creek, listen to my baby's pulse through my belly, and encourage Jonathan to try to hear the heartbeat through a stethoscope. They would gently feel with their hands and judge the welfare of both mother and child through their own intuitive processes. I felt loved and taken care of, part of an ancient tradition of wise women.

Only once during my pregnancy did I have to encounter the medical establishment. The midwives asked me if I would go and have blood work done at a local obstetrician's office. I called and made certain that they would do my blood work without having me as a prenatal client. I told them I had my own midwife and didn't need prenatal care from them, and they agreed. The blood work went fine, but when I went to pay my bill, the woman behind the counter said the doctor wanted to speak with me. I responded without thinking, "But I don't want to speak with the doctor." She looked desperately away from me to the doctor, who was out of my sight in the next room. She said, "But the doctor only wants to talk with you about the dangers of having a child at your age." My knees were knocking by this time, as my worst fears seemed to be turning into reality, and I was barely able to get myself out of the office without calling in my husband to rescue me.

I imagine most American women in the second half of the twentieth century would probably be happy to have a little talk with the doctor about the possible complications surrounding their baby's future birth. For me, it seemed like the kiss of death. I was already by that time quite phobic toward the medical establishment; I had been addicted to prescription drugs for ten years because of tension headaches and later developed an ulcer from having eaten so many pills for so many years. The doctors had never been able to help me, and they simply—by default, it seemed— kept giving me higher-dose (and higher-cost) prescriptions for heavier drugs. For some reason, the medications never helped with the headaches, but I was fast becoming a zombie as I depended on pills with names like meprobamate and Fiorinal several times each day. When I kicked the drug habit, I also kicked the Western medicine habit—cold turkey. I never wanted to have to deal with doctors again.

My midwife encouraged me to strengthen myself by hiking in the hills around my house. I used to climb a mound nearby, with stone ruins at the top, and then sit in trance looking down over the whole valley. Sometimes blue herons would dance in the sky over my head or stand calmly gazing in the creek below where I sat watching. At night, there were horned owls, and once during the winter, a golden eagle landed in a tree in our yard. During the late summer and early fall, the monsoons came to the desert. We would sit out on the porch and watch the storms coming across the desert, amazed at the beauty and power of nature's forceful daily spectacle. One early evening we were out walking on the cliffs overlooking the creek when a lightning storm moved quickly over the desert toward us. The lightning streaked horizontally across the entire expanse of desert sky, pitchfork-shaped, awesome to behold. Jonathan wisely thought that we should get off the hill and head for home. But I felt rushes of kundalini through my body, adrenaline and excitement expressing itself through my cells, and I couldn't relate to the danger.[2]

In that moment of cosmic connectedness to the forces of nature, I made a solemn vow to the Earth Mother. I gave us to her, for good. I said to her, "This baby and I belong to you completely. You may do with us what you wish." It was very dramatic and satisfying on a mythic level, and it seemed to anchor me in a profound state of trust. From that point on, I was not conflicted about medical intervention or riddled with fears about what might or might not happen with my birth. I simply put my trust in nature, and I allowed for the possibility of death. In so doing, I found my fears were eliminated and I could, from that point on, trust the process.

One day several months into my pregnancy, I got a tremendous craving for fish. We lived on beautiful Oak Creek in Arizona, so I decided I would catch a fish myself. I went to town and bought a fishing license and the necessary equipment, got worms for bait, and came home to try to remember how to fish. When I was a little girl, my father and grandfather had taken me fishing with them, but they had done all the dirty work for me. My need for the fish felt so instinctual, I knew it was the effect of my pregnancy. I wanted to honor it in a primal way, as a tribal or earth-based woman would have done. I marched myself down to the creek and prayed to the Mother of the Fish that I might catch just enough fish for me and my baby. The large catfish I caught practically jumped up out of the water. I got a rock and killed it in as sacred a way as I could, by clearing my mind and praying, and Jonathan cleaned and filleted it for dinner. I accompanied the fish with fresh cooked greens from our garden. I was never able to connect in that sacred way with the fish again, and I never caught another.

At one point during my pregnancy, I reexperienced the traumas connected with my earlier experiences of giving birth to my two daughters. I was reading a book about pregnancy as a therapeutic process, *Birthing Normally*, by Gayle Peterson, and it catalyzed a process of release for me that helped me move through the pregnancy in a healthy way. I remember walking out on the desert road, late at night in the dark, crying and crying as the visceral memories washed over me. I could smell the smells and see the paint in the hospital rooms, could feel which direction I had been lying in labor and remember all the details of what had been two fairly "normal" birthing experiences. With my first daughter, Robyn, in a modern teaching hospital in 1966, they called it "natural childbirth," by which they meant I could choose which anesthetic I wanted them to use. They induced my labor and broke my waters when my contractions stopped, even though I was three weeks early and they could have sent me home. And when Robyn spit up blood with her milk in the nursery, the doctor came in and gave me a shot to dry up my breasts. He said I had "abnormal" cells in my breast milk, and although he had no idea what that might mean (they didn't normally check women's milk so had no comparison), he felt I should not nurse. I was nineteen years old, and I didn't know I had any say in the matter.

My second daughter, Brooke, was born in a military hospital two years later. This time I knew I was a prisoner when I asked for water for my sore throat and they refused me. (They didn't want me to have to pee.) When I kept asking, because I had a cold and my scratchy throat needed that simple relief, the nurse came in with a large needle, and before I could stop her, inserted it into my buttocks. I was astonished. I asked what it was, and she said Demerol. I hardly remember anything else, except lying on the delivery table after the birth, falling asleep as the doctor sewed up my mandatory episiotomy, and hearing his voice as from a distance, saying, "Don't fall asleep, Mrs. Ziegler. We're almost finished." I didn't see my daughter until the next morning, which is several hours too late for the bonding instinct hormone to be released naturally from the brain. It took me years of conscious spiritual work to make up for what happened in that stupid, unnecessary assault on our primal experience together. Altogether, even with the intervention of a major tranquilizer, I was only in labor for two hours before Brooke was "delivered."

The reliving and release of traumatic earlier experiences are a part of what Gayle Peterson calls the organic "work of worrying" that a pregnant woman naturally does during her gestation period. The experiences, like all things held in the body, get stuck because a person has no way at the time to express a full range of feelings. I had never even let my entire experience of each birth come into full consciousness before. So as I walked on the road that particular night in Arizona, I felt my grief and rage as I had never known them, and I screamed to the black sky until I felt clean and clear.

One day toward the end of my pregnancy, my midwife felt the baby's position in my uterus and said, "The baby's lateral" (meaning laying sideways across the belly). "That's the worst position for birthing, and we're in the eighth month. You have to get him turned around!" I took her very seriously. That night in the bathtub, where I did my deep relaxation, I went into trance and told the baby just what the midwife had told me. "You have to get upside down, or we won't be able to birth at home." The next day, I had to teach a workshop in Los Angeles and had forgotten the incident in the bathtub. The baby was terribly restless, moving around and kicking, changing and shifting position, and I became concerned. Then suddenly I remembered the orders I had given him the night before, and I realized he was simply doing what I had asked. By the end of the day, he was shifted into proper place for birthing, with his head down, ready to drop into the passageway at birth time.

If Aaron Eagle had stayed in the "lateral" position and gotten too large to turn, I might have had to go to the hospital and might have "needed" a cesarean section. I hate to think what a doctor would have done, on noticing the lateral positioning of my child at the eight-month point. The midwife simply mentioned it to me, as she did everything she noticed. I had been reading *The Secret Life of the Unborn Child* by Thomas R. Verny, which discusses the child in the womb listening to music, hearing all the words, seeing all the pictures of the mother, experiencing everything happening around it.[3] When presented with the need for him to change position, it seemed perfectly natural to me that I would suggest the idea to him. I assumed that if he could hear and respond to us, then he could also make choices on his own behalf.

When my uterus prolapsed, one and a half weeks before I gave birth to Aaron at home, my midwife said it could be due to the use of forceps in my earlier births. Both my daughters had been delivered with forceps, for no good reason except that the technology existed. I must also be genetically predisposed to have problems in this area, because my mother, her mother, and one of my two sisters all have had a prolapsed uterus as well. All the daily walking I did during my pregnancy had toned my uterus very nicely, but nothing could repair the torn ligaments that were supposed to hold up the pelvic floor. The damage done to them almost twenty years earlier had come due.

I was very frightened, because I could feel my cervix from outside my vagina. It seemed like it might be the end of my dream to have a happy home birth. I had read about pregnant women being forced by the medical establishment to go to the hospital for birthing whether they wanted to or not. Court injunctions could make women have C-sections against their own wishes. I knew that at a certain point, my midwives might decide I was too high-risk. So I was pleasantly surprised when my midwife was relatively nonplused about my situation. She had "coincidentally" been trained by a master midwife whose own home birth at my age of thirty-seven involved a prolapsed uterus. She counseled us about what to expect and how to help, and we approached the birth with confidence.

I had to be prone in bed for a week and a half, while I waited for Aaron Eagle to emerge. My midwife had dreamed that he would be born quite early, and that everything would be all right. She always dreamed whatever complications were going to happen to a woman under her care, and that way she was prepared for the cord to be wrapped around a baby's neck, excess bleeding, a need for oxygen, or whatever. In my case, it was clear that the physical conditions were going to be fine, but there was something in the dream that showed her there would be a disappointment for me and Jonathan, which she couldn't understand at the time. She only mentioned this to us later, but when I went into labor three weeks before my due date, she wasn't worried about any of the physical conditions.

We had a wonderful birth experience, everything I had hoped for. In my case, it was true that the third time's the charm. Clearly a lot of the impetus for me to get pregnant with Aaron Eagle was so that I could complete the birth experience for myself the way it was meant to happen. I wanted to squat and have a baby, and I wanted to breast-feed. I felt cheated in relation to the botched experiences I had had, even though the results were my two wonderful, healthy girls. What woman in her right mind and healthy body would want to lie down on a metal table, put her feet up in stirrups, and have some male doctor remove the baby artificially from her body? Why on earth would she want her pubic hair shaved, sheets thrown over her blocking her view, and a surgical cut made from her vagina to her anus? It seems unbelievable to me now.

My birth was an initiation, just as it is for women in other cultures more earth-based than our own. I was transformed by it, as were the others who were able to be with us. In addition to my two wise women attendants and my husband, I was able to have my daughter (Brooke took photographs and cut the cord), my dear friend Karen Vogel, and our friend Hallie Austen, who had magically flown in from Berkeley for two nights. In tribal culture, birth is understood to be a doorway for women to gain empowerment through facing and overcoming obstacles and fear. Interfered with too much, as is the norm in Western culture, birth becomes a limiting experience in which we are unable to feel our own agency, with our natural courage and power. If I could have given birth naturally in my early twenties, I believe it would have made me a different woman.

Gayle Peterson's ideas about healing through pregnancy and birth were borne out the night we gave birth to Aaron. My daughter Brooke was living with Jonathan and me, going to high school in Cottonwood, Arizona. She had overcome her original urge to quit school when we first moved there and had successfully adapted to the country scene, becoming a pom-pom girl and all-around regular teenager. Still, she was the same girl who the summer before had read all of Mary Daly's *Gyn/Ecology*, no small task even for a grown woman, and she was able to understand and assimilate the profound feminist content of it. During my labor, when the midwife was taking a break from breathing with me and looking into my eyes, Brooke replaced her for a few moments, and she and I had a wondrous, healing experience. As we looked into each other's eyes, Brooke began to cry, and then so did I. I had chills all up and down my spine, and I said to her, "We've done this before, haven't we?" I knew in that moment that subtle things that had always been somehow unfinished were set right.

I started out my labor on all fours, because of the caution needed around the state of my uterus. Would it stay put? was the big question. But in that careful position, my cervix didn't dilate enough, and I finally decided I wanted to stand up. Jonathan stood like a tree, anchored to Mother Earth, and I stood and held onto him. It is without a doubt one of the best sharings we ever had. My cervix dilated appropriately, and finally my midwife said it was time to push. I didn't feel any urge to push, and I told her this, certain that my body would know when. A while later, she suggested more strongly that I needed to push now. Again I countered her advice, assuring her that my body would tell me when. She looked at me the way wise women stare

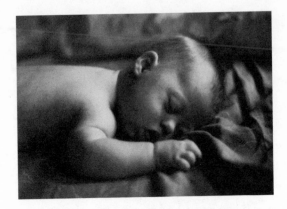

Aaron Eagle, one month old. Photo by Jonathan Tenney.

into the other world, and she said, "Now is the point when they used forceps. Your body doesn't know what to do. You need to push." That was all I needed; I pushed a few times (by now leaning back on the bed and clutching a large favorite crystal of mine), and Aaron Eagle came out.

Aaron was a little blue in that first minute of life. The telltale signs of his condition were, naturally, all present at the time of his emergence, but the midwives had the good grace to wait and see. I was completely innocent and didn't notice a thing, and if Jonathan knew, he did not mention it. (Later he told me he had dreamed that our baby had Down syndrome, but he didn't know whether or not to believe the dream.) I have deeply appreciated that blessed period of not-knowing. We were able to bond with Aaron completely, without the obstruction of a label, without knowing he had a "condition." There would be plenty of time to face that hurdle. We found his almond eyes very Asian and beautiful; his quiet serenity seemed to match his astrological chart—

Pisces Sun, Neptune-Moon conjunction in Capricorn—and we predicted he would be a little psychic boy.

All through my pregnancy, Jonathan had performed the functions of a model husband and father-to-be. He had rubbed my aching lower back and sacrum every single night before bed, lovingly giving of himself into this shared process of inventing Aaron Eagle. We used to sing together, lullabies, for Aaron Eagle in the womb.

> Tell me why the stars do shine,
> Tell me why the ivy twine,
> Tell me why the sky's so blue,
> And I will tell you why I love you.

> Because God made the stars to shine,
> Because She made the ivy twine,
> Because God made the sky so blue,
> Because She made you, that's why I love you.

But the tension between us as a couple had grown palpable, even though we were committed to not fighting during my pregnancy. I just couldn't handle the adrenaline that came with being upset or yelling and screaming. Two days after Aaron's birth, the tension erupted, and we had a horrendous fight in the bathroom. I remember my daughter Brooke's face as she left the house in horror. The fight was like an unfortunate oracle of what was to come for us, as we made the difficult descent from romance into "real life."

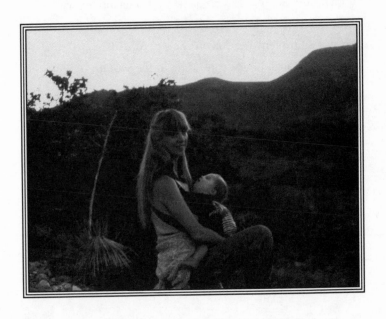

Vicki hiking with Aaron Eagle near their home
in Arizona. Photo by Jonathan Tenney.

Chapter Two

Instinctual Responses

༉

THE FIRST DAYS OF A CHILD'S LIFE ARE FELT TO be so precious and sacred for tribal societies that a new mother and child are cloistered behind closed doors, frequently in a place without light. This deliberately darkened, enclosed environment—clearly an extension of the womb— is maintained for varying lengths of time among different peoples, until the child is considered to be safe from harm and no longer in need of such an extreme form of protection. All mothers who birth at home must replicate this protocol in some respects, and certainly Aaron Eagle and I did. We rested in bed for a few days before becoming active and social. During this time, my main focus was on breast-feeding my new infant, and right away we had obstacles to face and overcome.

For some reason, Aaron had trouble with his eating. At first he seemed uninterested, and when I offered him the breast, he declined. My midwives encouraged me to relax and let Aaron find his own way, reminding me that all premature infants tend to have troubles of one kind or another. Since Aaron had been born more than three weeks before his delivery date, he fell into this category. There is a day or so prior to having milk when the only liquid in the breasts is "colostrum," a clear substance full of antibodies and very helpful to the immune system. They suggested that when the milk came in, he would probably be more interested. So we waited.

But when my milk came flooding in, and my breasts were engorged and ready to nurse, still Aaron Eagle seemed unable or unwilling to nurse. It was like a bad flashback for me, reminding me of what had felt like a personal failure to breast-feed my daughter twenty years earlier. I had been grief-stricken when the doctor said I couldn't nurse her, and I had had no one to talk to. The doctor's reference to "abnormal cells" haunted me for years, but I basically repressed the whole experience as I fed a bottle to my precious new daughter within the artificial limits of the hospital setting. No one around me at that time thought bottle-feeding was bad, and almost nobody else was breast-feeding anyway. My own mother had been able to breast-feed me for only a month before they told her she didn't have "enough milk."

Two years after Robyn's birth, when my daughter Brooke was born, I worked out privately, in a rather convoluted internal dialogue, the idea that if I tried nursing her and failed, it would feel terrible all over again; and if I tried and succeeded, my breast-feeding the second child might irreparably damage the self-esteem of the first one, who had been denied such a boon. At least this way my children would be equal. And now here I was fifteen years later, facing potentially the same kind of disappointment as before. Aaron Eagle was refusing to eat and growing steadily more listless. We had to act fast, as we were beginning to fear for his life.

Jonathan went out and bought a breast pump and an eyedropper. We pumped milk for Aaron, then dropped it into his mouth until he swallowed it. Like two parent birds feeding our little eaglet, we patiently and prayerfully got him to drink. I closed my eyes and used all my psychic will, crossing over some invisible barrier to his soul. I pulled on his life force, demanding that he live. Jonathan joined me in this silent prayer, and together we called to our son to respond. Little Aaron Eagle began to drink more of the precious liquid, slowly and mindfully learning to perform this animal task that all babies are supposed to know by heart.

One of those first nights, as I sat in bed with Aaron trying to nurse, with his daddy sleeping next to us, I felt frustrated at the ongoing difficulty we were having. He would suck for a few minutes, then lose the nipple and start to whimper. We did this over and over, until I felt I simply wouldn't be able to get it right. At that moment of hopelessness and despair,

I suddenly thought about La Leche League and all the breast-feeding mothers all over the world. Somewhere out there, sitting up alone in the dark in the middle of the night, was at least one other mother like me who was successfully feeding her child from her breasts. I began to draw on her energy, her knowledge, and consciously asked the La Leche League mothers of the world to lend me support, to reach out to me in the night and give me energy. I knew somehow if those other women could do it, so could I. My feeding came easier, as I became calmer and more centered.

It was much later, of course, that we learned that it is not uncharacteristic for babies with Down syndrome to have difficulties with nursing. They sometimes lack the normal sucking reflex of other babies, and they have to learn to suck by having their swallowing reflex stimulated. No doubt if we had been in a hospital, the staff would have switched us over to a bottle with a big enough nipple, and Aaron would have learned to swallow milk and then suck for it later. Once again, I would have missed out on the privilege of nursing my young. In our primal effort at getting Aaron to eat, we had stumbled on just the right solution to his problem, without having all the information. Our instinctual approach was perfect for establishing this patterning for Aaron, and he was gradually able to learn to breast-feed with great success.

It was through the labyrinth of the breast-feeding experience that we learned of Aaron Eagle's true "condition." Although we had very mixed feelings about taking Aaron to a doctor, the midwives had encouraged us to do just that, ostensibly because he was having so much trouble eating. Their hidden agenda, of course, was their suspicion that he might have Down syndrome. Without worrying us, they pushed for a medical diagnosis. We made an appointment for the local doctor to see Aaron six days after his birth, which happened to be Spring Equinox—one of the formal holidays of the ancient Goddess religion that we practiced. It is on this day that light and dark, day and night, are so perfectly and gravitationally balanced that it is said you can stand an egg on its end and it won't fall over.

On the sacred morning of Spring Equinox, I was sitting up with Aaron Eagle in my rocking chair; I had sat there all through that particularly difficult night. I thought as I sat and watched the dawn approach that this was as good a way as any to celebrate the ritual first day of spring. In that moment of first light, I experienced a profound sense of "visitation," and a voice seemed to advise me, "Be patient with this one." I rocked Aaron Eagle, imagining that I could sit up every night with him if need be. I felt an infinite sense of calm, a spaciousness that overrode my fatigue. I don't know why this presence from the spirit world was with me, but I felt grateful and content.

Suddenly there was a loud commotion outside the living room window. I turned to see one of our cats hanging by his front legs on the upper ledge of the window while his brother watched with interest from below. When Prince jumped down, I saw that he had a bird in his mouth, one of the lovely flycatchers that had been mating and nesting under the eaves of our adobe porch all that week. I felt terribly disturbed by this natural act of cruelty, wishing I hadn't witnessed it. And on a deeper level, I dreaded it as an ominous sign to have been shown to me on that sacred day.

The vision of the killed bird lingered with me throughout the day as I ran errands and prepared for Aaron's visit to the pediatrician. When we arrived at the doctor's office, nervous and ambivalent about being there, the nurse showed me, Jonathan, and Aaron Eagle to an examining room to wait for the doctor. Jonathan, my strong husband, looked ready to bolt, and I felt the same. There seemed to us to be a false sense of cordiality in the voices that greeted us there, the canned sound of professionals in a sterile, impersonal environment that looks at everyone in the same way. We felt alienated and disconnected. The nurse returned and took off Aaron's clothes in order to weigh him. She was not gentle or careful, as I would be. Neither was she rough or aggressive. She was simply indifferent to him as a person. She didn't conceptualize him as a perfect spirit in a tiny new body who might be overwhelmed or upset by brusqueness. While she acted as if nothing were wrong, we watched Aaron cry out loud for the first time in his life.

The doctor entered the room, wearing the aura of authority. He examined Aaron while we watched anxiously. This was the same doctor whose office had done my blood work during my pregnancy and who had wanted to "talk to me" about the dangers of having a child at my age. Of course, the very dangers he had been referring to had been realized, but I didn't know that yet. I suppose it makes a certain kind of logical sense that he remembered us and, from his point of view, felt vindicated that his prediction had been right. He didn't relate to our son; he simply handled him. And Aaron, who had never so far reacted negatively to anyone's touch, squirmed and complained. When he finished the examination, the doctor simply announced, "I think he has Down syndrome, but I can't be sure."

I felt myself go numb, and I heard my voice from a distance asking, "What does that mean?"

"Mongolism," he replied coldly. Pointing to different features on Aaron's face and mouth—his almond eyes, the folds of skin over the eye, his arched palate, his long tongue—he repeated what he had said already. He thought Aaron had Down syndrome, although he didn't have all the usual characteristics. For instance, the doctor pointed out that he didn't have a "simian line" across his palms, nor did he have a heart murmur, both typical features of the chromosomal abnormality. He advised us to have a blood test to find out for sure, which would cost us eight hundred dollars. When the doctor left the room, I started to cry, hearing my own inner voice telling me to "become like a crystal." We did not have the blood test done, and as we left the building, Jonathan cursed and promised that we would never go to another doctor.

I don't blame individual doctors and nurses for the ways they behave. My issues with the medical establishment are more general, going to the root of the very constructs of allopathic (Western chemical-based) medicine itself. I'd rather come at the problems of illness and disease from some other paradigm, such as Chinese medicine, for example. I once took Aaron to a Chinese herbalist for cold medicine, and in passing he mentioned to me that the Chinese had medicines "for this," he said, pointing to Aaron's eye folds, "and for this," pointing to some other feature on Aaron's face, and again "for this," pointing to his (then) sunken chest.

I was astounded. "You mean you can cure Down syndrome?" I asked in amazement.

"Down syndrome?" he asked, looking blank. "I don't know. But we can help this, and this, and this," he repeated, pointing to each part of Aaron's face and body that he had originally indicated. Apparently the Chinese don't even conceptualize Down syndrome as a "condition" that a person is stuck with. He looked at Aaron the same way he would look at you or me and had suggestions and potential solutions for what he perceived as a kidney weakness.

As we drove away from the doctor's office on that Spring Equinox in 1985, Jonathan and I felt our minds thrown open and a willingness to accept whatever would unfold. This spiritual expectation has stayed with us and more or less determined our direction with Aaron Eagle. As healers, our paradigm is one of service to humanity and, in a larger sense, service to those invisible forces of healing that underlie reality. Both Jonathan and I perceived ourselves as helpers in the world, with a mission to care and counsel. We saw the meaning of life's events written in the stars and felt our current situation to be an inevitable outcome of other lifetimes and experiences that had led to this moment in time.

This perception of ours is different from that disturbing New Age literalism that attaches blame and punishment to current experiences, saying that a person did something horrific in his or her last lifetime and that's why they got raped, murdered, or brutalized in this one; or that poverty and deprivation was determined by immoral or greedy acts in another time and place; or that we needed this burden to bear, because of some lesson we're learning, so we manifested a child with Down syndrome as a kind of terrible load to carry. These ideas are distortions of Eastern traditions brought through the Western filter of Christianity, with its blame and shame approach. Hinduism and Christianity are both patriarchal, judgmental, and hierarchical, and when you put them together it's a mess. "I'm bad, so I will go to hell," or "I was already bad or ignorant in the past, so I have to live in hell in this present lifetime."

I'm talking about a deeper, more ultimately Buddhist approach to life's everyday experiences and challenges. Buddhism, a religion of the East that is nonviolent and harmless toward all beings, constructs reality around the simple fact of human suffering and teaches that none of us can be free until everyone—all the people, animals, plants, and creatures of other realms—is free. I'm also speaking of a "shamanic call" and a deep, instinctual sense of personal destiny that is contained in the larger collective destiny of a time and place. Tribal peoples around the world live their lives from birth to death with this understanding of inclusion, containment, and personal calling. People with such a vision of life see themselves and the events in their lives as meaningful within their context, but they don't feel personally punished or rewarded by some God up there who's watching for mistakes.

So Jonathan and I felt expectant and "called" to the task of raising Aaron Eagle, although we had no concept of what this might mean. We brought him home from the doctor's office that day and began to relate to his condition in our own instinctual way. We invited friends in our rural community to come and visit us and meet this little being who had come to live with us. The people living alternative lifestyles in northern Arizona are a wonderful breed of human beings, and they created the perfect context for Aaron Eagle's arrival. These women and men had been spawned in the American sixties and were loyal to that "hippie" revolution, believing in a simple country life focused around children and going back to the land. Many of them had enormous organic gardens from which they satisfied most of their food needs; they built their own houses, created schools for their children, and healed themselves without chemicals or surgery. They were artists, midwives, farmers, architects, teachers, and masseuses. There was a health food store in town, a progressive preschool, and plenty of time taken for hiking, swimming, and generally appreciating the natural environment.

Jonathan and I had moved to this community while I was pregnant with Aaron Eagle, and we found our own niche there. As ritualists and alternative "ministers," we soon found ourselves leading community rituals on the Solstices and Equinoxes, gathering folks together for the communal sharing that ancient peoples practiced in relation to the Earth Mother and the cycle of changing seasons. The women had read my book *Motherpeace* and gathered around me to learn Motherpeace Tarot and esoteric healing. We practiced our personal brand of Goddess religion on the four cross-quarter holidays, February 1st (Candlemas), May 1st (Beltane), August 1st (Lammas), and November 1st (Hallowmas), and our circle grew in strength and numbers. We bonded, not only as friends, but as a community of like-minded people.

We received back from this tribe a reflection of Aaron Eagle as beautiful, wondrous, and a certain blessing to us. It was just what we needed. Their reactions to Aaron affirmed and sanctified our own impression of his loveliness, his ethereal, fairylike specialness. There was no one in our immediate circle to suggest that there was anything wrong with him, or with us for having him. Nobody told us to get tests or further diagnoses; all responses to his arrival were of unconditional welcome. People came with gifts and blessings, wishing us well, letting us know they were there in our lives with whatever needs we might have. Clearly, they believed in us. Without minimizing the challenge that we would have to face, they considered us able to do it. We needed this reflection of strength and possibility, the belief that we had what it would take to raise Aaron Eagle well.

My own midwestern family got a chance to respond to Aaron Eagle in the first two weeks of his life, as well. My mother and her parents drove to Phoenix and stopped on their way, while I was still pregnant with Aaron. A week after his birth, on their return trip to Iowa, they stopped again to visit and welcome our new baby. They arrived two days after we learned about Aaron's condition. When they came in the house, I told them the story and showed them the baby. They were shocked, but careful and loving, shedding a few tears and providing tremendous support. We carried on in a normal way for a few hours, all of us doing the best we could to respond well to such a devastating situation. If having a child with Down syndrome is considered a tragic and sorrowful event in our culture, then naturally this sense of suffering spreads into the family's community of friends and relatives. This potential grief is very confusing, becoming a source of ambivalence, fragmentation, uncertainty, depression, anger, and tension.

I've already spoken about the expectation in our household that any child to whom Jonathan and I gave birth would be in some way "special," and that we accepted Aaron's diagnosis as a fateful gift to us from the Divine. We saw each other as larger-than-life romantic partners, and we infused our marriage with this notion of destiny. Our refuge was in being with the child himself, so sweet, so angelic, his little eyes so soft, his helplessness demanding our protection and love. "Be more patient with this one," the voice had whispered to me. Aaron's condition was a Mystery that gave rise to awe in us.

After dinner that night, my mother and I were alone for a while in the kitchen, doing the dishes and having a moment together. She and I had been through every kind of shift in our relationship over the years, as I had found my way into feminism, bisexuality, and other lifestyle differences. It wasn't always easy for the two of us to connect, and although we maintained a love for each other under everything, I know we both felt alienated at times. During my spiritual awakening in the late seventies, I had made my own necessary separation from my mother, not seeing her (or anyone in my biological family) for a few years while I lived as an artist in Berkeley, creating the Motherpeace cards. I had to process the fact that my family back in Iowa couldn't really understand me, and that maybe they wouldn't ever really know me. I had to find the strength in myself to validate my own identity and path in the world, whether they accepted me or not.

But my mother was a card player herself, and there was a place in her that could recognize the Tarot as something other than a threat. When she finally visited me in Berkeley in the late 1970s, I read her cards, and she loved it. After all, I reminded her, she was the person in my early life who taught me to wish on white horses, wishing stars, and four-leaf clovers. I've always attributed my easy connection to nature-magic in part to her unconscious impulses in that direction. Whenever I shuffle the round Motherpeace Tarot cards, I feel my mother's presence at the table, her imprint on me from all those late card nights in my early upbringing. My mother always had a bridge club, and when we went to Lake Okiboji every summer with my grandparents and aunts and uncles, we played poker for pennies on those rainy afternoons when we couldn't fish or sunbathe.

So that night, in my Arizona kitchen, we were in a somber mood as we washed the dinner dishes together. It was certainly a relief to my family that I had got myself married again to a man and had this baby. At least we had something normal to discuss, an undisputed common ground between us. My mother and I suddenly turned toward each other, and we both started to cry. I suppose we had both been keeping a stiff upper lip, as is our practice, and in that moment the tension resolved itself into spontaneous tears that shook through our defenses against pain and vulnerability. We hugged each other, and my mother said to me from her heart, "You're the only one in our family who could have handled this, Vicki."

I had never felt so fully seen, affirmed, and valued by my mother before that moment. I had never understood that she could perceive who I was beyond our external differences and disagreements. At the age of thirty-seven, I felt for the first time accepted unconditionally by my mother. I'm not saying that she didn't love me before that, just that I was not able to realize it fully. And perhaps neither was she. It's hard to accept a child who is different in some way, as I was when I was growing up, and as Aaron Eagle would be. I liked being different, but on the other hand, I suffered the fate of all artists and iconoclasts, which is to feel quite isolated inside from the thoughts and behavior and values of those around me. I was always desperately seeking to be understood, yet defying the cultural norms, and I frequently felt rejected or misunderstood instead. In that cathartic moment in the kitchen, I saw that without having an academic understanding of shamanism or tribal medicine, my mother understood that I am a healer.

After my family went back to Iowa, we sent birth announcements to everyone in our larger circle telling of Aaron's arrival. How do you say it? "We are happy to announce the birth of our long-awaited little boy, and oh, by the way, he has something wrong with him . . ." I sat for days and painstakingly handwrote every announcement, telling all our friends and relatives in my own words exactly what seemed to be the truth. Aaron had a condition that meant that he would be developmentally delayed and never be normal, and that we loved and appreciated him enormously and felt his presence in our life as a blessing that we hoped they would share and celebrate with us.

When we began to receive cards and letters back to us, the loving response they contained was overwhelming. People rose to the occasion, responding exactly as we had hoped. They repeated my mother's assurance that Jonathan and I could handle it, that Aaron Eagle was lucky to have us for parents, and that we would fulfill ourselves. People shared stories with us and sent pictures of other "retarded" children they had known who had brought happiness into the lives of their families. Many people told me they deeply appreciated the words I had written to let them know and the way I had shared myself so directly with them. I couldn't really remember what I had said, just that I had opened my heart and let the words spill out as they wished.

Someone sent me a copy of Barry Kaufman's *Son-Rise,* the awe-inspiring story of an autistic boy whose parents organized themselves around the task of breaking through to him and succeeded in extraordinary ways, bringing about a transformation of his illness and its "normal" development. I began to read everything I could get my hands on about Down syndrome and other forms of mental disability. Jonathan went to the Phoenix public library and came home with a copy of *The World of Nigel Hunt,* a true story of a boy with Down syndrome written by Nigel Hunt himself as a young adult! He told all about his own process, in conscious comparison with the worries and fears of his parents on his behalf. It was funny, direct, and not at all self-conscious or embarrassing. Similar to it is the recently published *Nobody Nowhere,* a brilliant autobiographical story by Donna Williams, who discovered she was autistic at the age of twenty-five and has been able to write and speak about it publicly, illuminating the condition by articulating it from the inside![1]

We began to reach for hope, to build an exciting, larger-than-life story about Aaron that would measure up to our own fantasies and expectations of ourselves. Yes, he had Down syndrome, but there were articles about miracle cures, methods of "bridging" past the damage so that he would be able to read and write with the best of us.[2] Surely, if any couple could push their retarded child past what was ordinarily anticipated, it would be the two of us! We became a devoted and dedicated team of parental coaches, cheering Aaron from the sidelines of his life.

In the literature we first read, it said that one common response to giving birth to a child with Down syndrome is denial. "This cannot be happening to me, to my child, to our family."[3] Parents think it won't be like they say, and that something unusual will intervene and change everything for the better. Denial tends to progress toward anger and fear, and finally guilt. What did we do wrong? What drug, pill, or X ray caused the fatal flaw in our chromosomes? Was it his mother or his father who was to blame? (They used to blame the mother's "old eggs" for Down syndrome; now they say that in at least 25 percent of the cases, the "fault" lies with the father's genetic makeup.)[4] Parents of disabled children generally feel all these feelings, not necessarily in that order, at one time or another.

I worked very hard to get in touch with my emotions about Aaron and to be truthful about my feelings in relation to him and his condition. I struggled to stay awake in the face of the confusion of holding the enormous paradoxical reality that parents of a handicapped child have to contend with. On the one hand, there was our beautiful new baby boy, responding and interacting with us in his admittedly limited ways, but responding nonetheless. And we loved him and adored him, fiercely. Wasn't he truly beautiful, or were we making that up? Did he look funny to other people, and were they kind enough not to mention it? We lost perspective and couldn't tell at times. Then there was the cultural reality of the label describing him: a person with Down syndrome, retarded, disabled.

I was angry all right, but for a long time, it wasn't anger at Aaron or at the universe. I felt a fury at our conditioning process, the cultural naming activity that erases diversity and wants homogeneity above all else. Some stranger would say, "Oh that's too bad," in response to being told about Aaron Eagle, and I wanted to scream at them, "No it isn't! Can't you see, he's perfect the way he is?" I couldn't see how I would ever be able to reconcile the pleasure I took in our private experiences of nursing, rocking, and singing with the way the outside world viewed Aaron and our "tragedy." I felt trapped in other people's pictures, afraid I would never get free. He seemed like such a wonderful boy; I wanted people to look past his disability and see his soul inside. We discussed other countries we might move to, where people with Down syndrome are more accepted, less stigmatized. Switzerland. China. Just somewhere else.

Finally, just before Fall Equinox almost six months later, I was walking up in the foothills above our home, and I suddenly felt integrated. I didn't know why it happened, but I felt free of the conflict that had been working its way out in me all those early months. I thought of how creative I am and how I get bored easily and need to change my activities often. I thought about how I had already raised two children to adulthood, that I knew how to do that. If Aaron Eagle had been another normal child, I might have been bored or distracted, might have felt that I could be doing something better or more important than raising him. Instead, I felt both called and qualified to be his mother. I knew I would always be stimulated, never bored, with the challenges he would present to me through the painful and paradoxical reality of his condition. I had a mission.

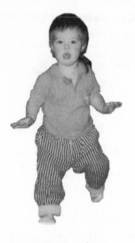

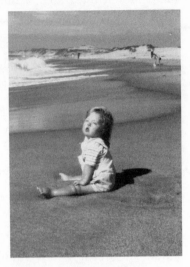

Aaron Eagle taking
his first steps in the
Salt Lake City
Airport, age two.
Photo by author.

Aaron Eagle's first visit to
the Pacific Ocean,
age fourteen months.

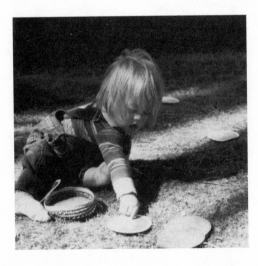

Aaron Eagle
playing with
Motherpeace Tarot
Cards in Santa
Cruz. Photos by
Jonathan Tenney.

Chapter Three

Energy Medicine

৵

AARON'S FIRST REAL HEALTH CRISIS OCCURRED when we introduced solid foods into his diet. When he was four months old, we toured the country, stopping in Minneapolis, Denver, Salt Lake City, and Northern California, where I taught workshops, using the Motherpeace images I had created with my friend Karen Vogel. Jonathan drove the car, entertained Aaron, and brought him to me during breaks for breast-feeding. We started to notice a strange phenomenon whenever we would go into a restaurant to eat a meal. Aaron made funny noises, like he was agitated or upset. Could it be he was hungry for food? I had read all the New-Age baby books, and I didn't intend to add solid food to his menu until he was nine months old! Finally, out of curiosity and a kind of disbelief that has come to feel familiar in relation to Aaron, we tried giving him some baked potato one night. He loved it. He couldn't get enough. He smacked his lips and hummed for more. I started him on natural cereals. A friend suggested sweet potato. He even sucked on pickled ginger in a Japanese sushi restaurant. He seemed to like almost everything we introduced.

Although he strongly desired to eat, he seemed unable to process the solid food by having normal bowel movements. I tried psyllium husks and other natural laxative foods, but he stayed pretty much stuck, causing him to get a stomach ache and cry inconsolably. This blockage in his intestinal system was very frightening for me and Jonathan, and we quickly learned how to give Aaron enemas in a warm bathtub in order to bring him relief in his elimination process.

Around the same time, we were given an article written in 1980 by Dr. Henry Turkel, the Austrian-American inventor of bone marrow infusion and biopsy instruments used in this country and throughout the world. Dr. Turkel has treated patients with Down syndrome since 1940, using nutritive ("orthomolecular") as well as medical approaches, especially the "U Series" treatment he developed, which "combines hormones, antihistamines and other medications, and nutrients that act as coenzymes in the body."[1]

The amazing approach Dr. Turkel takes is that Down syndrome is primarily an elimination disease, a "storage disease," as he calls it. Due to the presence of the extra chromosome, tissues clog with minerals, fats, and fluids, which can be reduced through megavitamin and enzyme therapy. The otherwise sluggish elimination system leads to deterioration of brain cells and more retardation as the person ages. The article included remarkable pictures of children who had made notable improvements over time under his program. Their stooped, stodgy figures changed to lean, taller children's bodies as they progressed with the diet he recommended.

This simple but unorthodox treatment, which includes such substances as vitamin C and digestive enzymes, showed "improved general health, physical development, and mental function" for patients in the United States from 1952, and he has documented its use in Europe. It is highly recommended by Glenn Doman and the Institutes for Human Potential in Philadelphia. But the Food and Drug Administration forcibly suppressed the information and the use of this treatment for Down syndrome in this country for twenty-five years. "The AMA, hospitals, research institutions are all included in the list of those industries that fear the economic threat of our greater independence from drugs and hospitalization." Turkel notes that one specific combination of the series was designated "unscientific" by the FDA and then later marketed by two drug companies with FDA approval. A 1988 article on Turkel in *East/West Journal* says that he has finally won approval for use of the U Series in Michigan, where he practices.[2]

Understanding Dr. Turkel's theory helped Jonathan and me in our approach to Aaron Eagle's elimination difficulties.

We treated the symptoms as warnings of an underlying structural problem, and we have since been very careful with his intake of anything that might be undigestible or hard to assimilate. This means as little white bread and pasta as possible (using whole wheat instead), no refined sugar (substituting honey, malt syrup, maple syrup, fruit juices, etc.), and as many good fibrous foods as he will eat to help his intestines to move and to avoid blockages. Brown rice is especially helpful in this regard, as are all other whole grains and fresh vegetables. We make a supreme effort to get organic or unsprayed foods for Aaron Eagle, so that he will not be subjected to pesticides and other poisons, which build up in the system (for everyone) and cause more trouble with digestion and assimilation.

At the time we had problems with Aaron Eagle's eating and elimination, we heard from friends about a Japanese woman healer in Phoenix only two hours from where we were living. Mary Burmeister is the Master teacher of Jin Shin Jyitso in the United States. We took Aaron Eagle, at seven months old, to visit her, and she saw him free in between her paying clients. This meant we had a total of about five minutes of her time at each visit, yet with a focused, delicate touch she created absolutely extraordinary results. Aaron was immediately calmer and happier after each treatment. She showed Jonathan how to do what she did (he took a few classes from her after that), and he began to do simple hands-on healing for Aaron every day. Within only one week of this hands-on work, Aaron started having easy, regular bowel movements, without the need of any special foods or supplements or other attention. His energy field cleared so much that he looked physically different. His eyes were brighter and clearer, he was happier, he learned better, and he made the effort to communicate more.

In the United States, it is customary for people to use exclusively Western medical approaches to our health, and alternative methods are often viewed with alarm by the mainstream. Parents are indoctrinated about the necessity of performing only certain "acceptable" procedures upon our children from birth. Even giving birth at home, as we had done with Aaron Eagle, is considered deviant; only one percent of all birthing happens at home anymore. Concomitant with this deeply held trust in allopathic medicine is a strong suspicion that arises in opposition to any invisible or "paranormal" methods of healing, such as hands-on, faith healing, or "energy medicine." Yet Jonathan and I have always found these methods to be the most effective with Aaron Eagle, and we feel grateful for having been introduced to Asian and other so-called alternative ways of healing, as well as eating.

One of the main problems faced by parents is the tendency for some children with Down syndrome to "become obese as they grow older."[3] Aaron's first special education teacher told us that, in her experience, children with Down syndrome find it hard to stop eating, as if they have no natural limits on their appetites. She warned us we would need to carefully watch for this tendency in Aaron from an early age in order to keep him healthy and fit. But Aaron has never shown a tendency to eat the addictive foods that lack nutrition, and the foods he does eat, which are healthy, seem to fill him up without making him fat. Certainly, he has a healthy appetite and often eats a lot, but even now he eats mainly brown rice, granola, organic eggs, whole wheat breads, peanut butter, plain yogurt, and fruits.

The salient point here is that Aaron has never developed a taste for sugar. White, refined sugar is the most harmful of the addictive foods, and I believe it is an unnatural taste that must be cultivated. If you give babies ordinary baby food in jars, it has so much sugar and salt in it that they become addicted to it early on. But when Aaron was a baby, we never presented him with sugared foods; we always offered him plain or honey-sweetened items instead. He therefore never seemed to need sugar or even be attracted to it, and he almost always avoids it now by choice. I once watched a little girl offer him a powdered-sugar doughnut from a box, which he eagerly tasted and then quickly returned to the giver. I will sometimes get him a cookie from a bakery near home, but he never eats more than half of it. The sugary sweetness is just more than he needs, having never become chemically addicted to it.

If "you are what you eat," then whatever food goes into Aaron's body has a lot to do with his health, or lack of it. I think of food as medicine, nature's way of providing what the body needs to thrive. Our way of doctoring Aaron has been mainly preventive, starting with natural, or organic, unprocessed ingredients in his food. The Japanese have found that foods like miso soup and brown rice actually reduce levels of radiation in the body, and honey has measurable medicinal benefits as well. Since we understand his elimination to be a central key to Aaron's health, we take it very seriously. It is interesting too that so far Aaron generally refuses to eat meat. We got some chicken down him once, but he came home and threw it up shortly afterward. He seems to prefer to be a vegetarian. He is more of a purist than either his dad or I. No fish, no meat, period.

Once, when Aaron was a baby, he got a high fever and stopped eating for days. Since fever is the body's way of cleansing itself, we didn't want to take it away from him. But we didn't want him to wither away, either. After a couple of days, Jonathan and I did everything we could think of to coax him into taking a bite of something. Finally, after three days, reluctantly, but instinctively, we force-fed him the liquid from cooked split peas. He became well almost immediately after eating a small amount of this protein-rich food. Once we got him eating something, then he was willing (as if he remembered how) to do it for himself. It seems he had just gotten stuck in the noneating mode.

I don't expect that everyone who reads this will be interested in how to use preventive and alternative methods in raising a child with Down syndrome. But for those who do have an interest, it is crucial to find support and avoid isolation. Avoiding the usual interventions from doctors, chemicals, and medical technology is difficult on your own, and parents need support and discussion with other parents within a holistic framework. In a culture that is not rooted in earth-based methods and approaches, one must learn new (ancient) information and methods to replace the Western system. A strong motivation has to be there in the parents, since it means at times bucking the system and going against the general consensus.

Natural medicine can take longer, in general, to effect a cure, but the cure is deeper and more thorough in the long run. It takes faith and patience to let symptoms, such as fever, do their work without trying to make them go away. Every step of our way with Aaron Eagle has been a confirmation of the natural methods versus Western chemical or technological ones. For that reason, I want to try to elucidate the madness in our method of approach to his care, which is rooted in the ancient Goddess tradition of Old Europe.

During the Middle Ages, the methods and remedies used by the so-called witches (women healers) in Europe were appropriated and written down by male scholars who had access to the newly-invented Gutenberg printing press. Traditional midwives and healers were systematically eradicated from their communities by the power of the Catholic Inquisition. The four centuries from the 1200s to the 1600s have come to be known as the Burning Times, because an estimated nine million women healers were tortured and burned at the stake for the crime of having the power to cure.[4] These women shamans were annihilated, along with their especially feminine, intuitive approaches to illness and healing; however, their herbal remedies and their medicinal ways were actually systematized into what later became obstetrics, gynecology, and pediatrics. The tribal base of Old European medicine was lost, and the "cures" were codified into formulas and extracts that are still used today (in synthetic forms) in modern pharmacology. Unfortunately, when an element from nature is extracted and used by itself, rather than in conjunction with the other chemical portions of the plant—bark, stem, leaf, or root—it is more dangerous. Modern medicines, for this reason, have more unexpected and deleterious side effects.

In raising my daughters during the 1970s, I used as many natural methods as I was able to transmit to them, and they have both learned to manage their health through these alternative approaches. With a "special" child like Aaron Eagle, this approach is even more challenging, since he can't usually describe his ailment, isn't as responsive in his nerve endings as a normal child, and balks at foul-tasting herbs or strong treatments. We have recently experienced a brilliant success in this department, as I acquired some liquid vitamin B from the Institutes for Human Potential in Philadelphia and brought it home to Aaron Eagle, who has never before been willing to take any vitamins, not even the cute little dinosaurs they make for kids. I announced to him that this was going to make him feel so good that he was going to be asking me for it, saying, "Mommy, Mommy, give me my B!" I was teasing him, but

I must have inadvertently used some hypnotic technique, because every single day since then, twice a day without fail, Aaron Eagle the clown gets my attention and shouts, "Mommy, Mommy, Mommy, give me my B!" and then swallows the rather bad-tasting liquid with only a grimace, following it with a glass of juice.

One of the problems facing parents of special children is that so many of the kids are born with physical problems that require medical intervention from the beginning of their lives. Things like holes in the valves of the heart, heart murmurs, fluids in the ear, and so on are common, with up to half of the children with Down syndrome having something seriously wrong. Parents are naturally terrified when told by the presiding physician that their child might not live without the surgery or drugs that are being recommended. How do we know how to make informed decisions about the health of our special children? Where do we draw the line between being responsible and overintervening? How do we learn about other effective ways of healing and preventing illness so that we are not totally dependent on the chemical and surgical techniques that Western medicine is so good at?

We took Aaron on his first long trip to the East Coast when he was still a baby. Jonathan and I were teaching workshops during the day and staying with strangers at night. Aaron was supposed to go to sleep in a crib set up for him in the room where we were sleeping. For hours, he was unable to sleep. He didn't cry and wasn't in pain but seemed "wired" and nervous, making repetitive sounds and banging his face on the pillow. We tried all kinds of approaches, patting him and singing, trying to lull him into sleep. Suddenly, somewhere in the middle of the night, tired and in a somewhat altered state myself, I thought of burning sage.

Native American people burn sage (what they call "smudging") to rid the house and the psychic field of invading forces that could harm a person or a place. I had brought sage along on the trip because of the classes I was teaching on healing, but I hadn't thought to use it for our family. No wonder tribal people are always perplexed at the Western tendency to split off the sacred from the "mundane"! I lit the sage and blew some in Aaron's direction, and within about three minutes he had fallen peacefully asleep. Whatever beings or energies were keeping him awake must have cleared out very quickly when confronted with this age-old Native American purification remedy. The particular presences on this night were benign but keeping Aaron awake, which was inconvenient for all of us.

In the shamanic view it is not primarily germs, but also negative vibrations and even "entities" that create illness by coming unbidden into the body of the sick person. It is understood by shamanic people that forces of illness hang around and invade our bodies, causing us no end of trouble. The few times that Aaron has come down with something, it seemed to fall within this framework of illness. In tribal culture, shamans are called in to diagnose the problem by finding out which negative energies are present, what they want, and how to get rid of them. In different cultures, healers use different techniques of expelling—sucking, blowing, fanning, scanning with an egg or a guinea pig, using the hands or a crystal, drumming, smoking, even straightforward negotiation. But always, they get rid of the invading "demon" responsible for the illness and retrieve the soul, which may have inadvertently left the body.

I had to take Aaron with me one day to take care of some business forty-five minutes away from home with a group of women who harvested and made formulas from natural flowers and herbs, creating essential oils for healing. When we walked into the apartment, the atmosphere felt kind of "thick" to me, but I ignored it and proceeded to make my purchase. Within a few minutes, Aaron became violently ill. He had a raging fever, his face became red and patchy, he seemed to be breaking out in a rash of some kind on his body, and I was sure he must be getting the measles. I rushed us out of there. But as soon as we were in the car on the highway for home, Aaron became completely well. It was shocking. He didn't have any symptoms at all by the time we had been driving for fifteen minutes.

Now I suppose Aaron could have been having an allergic response to some physical substance in the environment of which I was not aware. But one of the things that frequently happens in "possession illnesses" is that the body burns up the problem through a high fever. Buddhism says

the body burns the karma, freeing the person of the affliction. Buddhists and shamans understand that healers often
burn up karma for others, in a voluntary sacrificial act. I
wonder if Aaron didn't burn up somebody's karmic goo
that day and leave the place cleaner than when we arrived.
But how would I have explained that to a medical person?

Western medicine considers people with Down syndrome to need more, not less, medical intervention than others, and the medical establishment projects onto parents like
Jonathan and me that we are "irresponsible" and unpardon-
ably defiant in our attitudes. Our approach is so different,
they think we're crazy. For example, we have not immunized Aaron Eagle, and we hope we don't ever have to. But
that decision was not made casually. Part of the reading I did
during my pregnancy convinced me that immunizations are
an incorrect way of approaching the protection of children.[5]
One of the most disturbing things that research has turned
up is the statistical link between sudden infant death syndrome (SIDS or "crib death") and inoculations. Americans
think we are protecting our three-month-old infants with
their compulsory DPT shots, but we may be killing some ten
thousand of them every year. My own daughter Robyn suffered the typical "inexplicable" high fever and convulsions
that are characteristic of the reactions to DPT shots. Many
of the crib deaths take place within a short time after the
visit to the doctor. I've personally heard someone who knew
a crib death child say, "She was feeling fine. In fact, she had
just had her checkup at the doctor's the other day!"

Jonathan and I have studied and pondered the problem for years, and it looks to us as though there is enough hard evidence showing immunizations to have serious risks that it is our informed decision to prevent Aaron from getting DPT or other childhood vaccinations. This decision of ours always causes a certain amount of trouble when we want to send Aaron to school or day care. This subject is so complex that any parent who delves into it must then struggle with the potential choices. Thanks to the many court battles fought by the Christian Scientists over the years, we have the right to refuse to have Aaron vaccinated. But if Aaron is not immunized, will he be able to safely travel in foreign countries? And once when he was in kindergarten, there was a measles scare at school. We were told Aaron couldn't attend school until the potential epidemic had passed—possibly for three months—unless we gave him a measles shot. The schools may not have the right to insist that we come with our vaccination card, but apparently they can keep our child from actually attending school in an "emergency." It turned out not to be measles that day, so the problem didn't have to be resolved. It remains to be seen whether we will be allowed to practice our beliefs in this area and keep Aaron enrolled at school.

I remember my first confrontation around this issue. When Aaron was a year old, we moved back to California. After a whole summer of finding housing, getting settled, and beginning our private practices as healers, we entered into the process of enrolling Aaron in a school or day care program. I had to do a phone interview with someone from the Regional Center in Alameda County, who questioned me about a doctor for Aaron. I said he didn't have a doctor. The intake person said, "Where does he go when he's sick?" And I answered, truthfully at that time, "Well, he hasn't really been sick." She gasped and warned, "Well, you've been lucky!" And I laughed and said, "No, we've been really careful."

In *Confessions of a Medical Heretic*, written in 1980, Dr. Robert Mendelsohn says that his (then) twenty-five years as a practicing physician convinced him that "Annual physician examinations are a health risk; hospitals are dangerous places for the sick; most operations do little good and many do harm; medical testing laboratories are scandalously inaccurate; many drugs cause more problems than they cure; the X-ray machine is the most pervasive and most dangerous tool in the doctor's office."[6]

It may be true that many children with Down syndrome seem to have a greater number of colds and ear infections than other kids. When I say that Aaron has never had an ear infection, I feel like knocking on wood! But the common medical treatments of inserting tubes in the ears and prescribing routine antibiotics for strep throat, for example, seem quite inappropriate, in my mind, to a growing child's constitution.

Again I quote Dr. Mendelsohn, this time from his later book, *Male Practice: How Doctors Manipulate Women:* "It is riskier than Las Vegas to take your child to a pediatrician for treatment of an earache or a mild sore throat."[7] He goes on to detail the high incidence of needless tonsillectomies that were performed in this country before 1965 as what he calls "bread and butter" surgeries, the kind that keep doctors in ready income. When the medical evidence against tonsillectomies became overwhelming, the surgeries decreased, only to be replaced with "tympanostomy," a procedure in which "small tubes are inserted through the eardrums to drain the middle ear of children suffering from an infection. . . . It is supposed to prevent hearing loss, but studies indicate not only that it doesn't, but that the operation itself does in some children produce scarring that causes hearing loss."[8] Putting tubes in the ears is still a very common treatment for children who have Down syndrome, since they are believed to be more susceptible than normal children to ear infection and hearing loss.

Similarly, synthesized antibiotics depress the immune system and prevent it from operating at full capacity. I have heard alternative healers make a correlation between antibiotic treatments and systemic yeast, or candida, which makes sense since every woman who has ever taken antibiotics knows that a yeast infection often follows. With so many people suffering from these afflictions these days, it pays to explore these associations and to find other ways of treating illness. Healers from the Middle Ages knew the healing secret of garlic—used fresh and taken regularly. Garlic is nature's natural antibiotic, killing only harmful bacteria, unlike artificial antibiotics, which kill off all the flora and fauna in the body that are necessary to its healthy functioning. Garlic seems to provide a natural boost for the immune system. After eating raw garlic every night for a week, a person will find that strep throat or even pneumonia is gone but all the necessary bacteria in the body are still present, doing their proper job, without causing a yeast infection. Garlic can even get rid of worms and *Giardia* without medical intervention. Even though I know this from my own experience, as well as my research, it's practically against the law for me to make such a statement. Yet I have personally relied on garlic for getting well when I'm sick for almost twenty years now.

Like Christian Scientists, who pray over their children and ask for divine intervention in the problems of disease and illness, we have always "channeled" healing power for Aaron. The shamanic or "earth-based" approach that we favor is active, requiring someone to clear the "aura" or field, and in serious cases, the patient needs to ingest something herbal or have body work or acupuncture. For example, when Aaron has a cold or flu, I rub garlic oil from the local health food store on the bottoms of his feet, put wool socks under his jammies, and send him to bed. The garlic is absorbed readily into his system through his feet, and with a little vitamin C in his juice, he gets well in a very short time. He has never taken any other kind of antibiotics or drugs.

Even when I was still nursing Aaron, this issue came up indirectly when I got an infected tooth and my dentist said

I would need surgery. I've had wisdom teeth removed in the past, and I remembered the strong anesthetic. I was unwilling to subject Aaron as an infant to the chemicals, and I certainly didn't want to stop breast-feeding. The dentist argued with me until I got upset and told him that I was nursing a retarded child, and I absolutely wasn't going to have the surgery at that time, no matter what. His heart opened, and he completely changed his tune, telling me what I could do instead! I was to use hydrogen peroxide and a syringe, which he gave me, to clean out the infected tooth. He didn't really trust it would work, but without other options, he informed me of this older tried-and-true method. It worked in a matter of days, and I have never had trouble with the tooth again. I wish I were privy to other supposedly outdated methods for healing disease, those that predate the too-easy surgery we have today!

The medical establishment has bullied many parents into being afraid for our children's health, and we often develop a distorted sense of what it means to be "responsible." To me, medicine looks like our national religion, with the white-coated doctors as priests. Why do people defend doctors so strongly? Why is it so terribly upsetting to almost everyone when I say that Aaron doesn't have a pediatrician, and that we don't want one? It's treated almost as blasphemy. Like other persecuted groups, we who prefer alternative medicine want the right to practice our own way of healing. The accumulated medical dogma that is taught as fact in medical schools comes from research funded by drug companies and promoted by the American Medical Association. It is not unbiased. Funding is unceremoniously cut off when a researcher discovers a cure as simple, natural, and cheap as echinacea, golden seal, or vitamin C. Natural, organic remedies are referred to as "quackery."

I know we're all conditioned by these strong cultural beliefs, because even I still come under their influence at times. As embarrassing as it is to me, with my alternative position, I have occasionally become overwhelmed and afraid about illness, and once I even took Aaron to the emergency room. Doing so only served to renew my commitment to the natural approaches, however, at the same time that it showed me how strong America's reliance on the medical system can be. If I don't even believe in Western medicine and don't have health insurance, and still I ran to the emergency room, surely others must also use it at times when it is not necessary.

It happened one evening around dinnertime, as I was bringing Aaron home from day care. We were walking up the front steps of our house, when he kind of gasped and doubled over, becoming suddenly ill. Rather than approach the problem shamanically, I fell blindly into the fears of an American mother for her child. He was breathing funny and holding his stomach, crying, and trembling. I was ungrounded and I panicked. Once we were inside the house, it got worse. I have always said I would go to a doctor for a broken leg or a car accident, or any other clear-cut physical problems that they know how to cure. In this case, I was

convinced that he must have either appendicitis or poison-
ing, and both seemed like things that could be handled better by doctors. I bundled him into the car and off to
Children's Hospital. When we got there, we had to wait
and wait for an exam. Aaron was listless and pale. The
waiting room was full of children who potentially had
measles and other communicable diseases, so they quaran-
tined Aaron and me in a small isolated room, ostensibly to
protect him, since he has not been inoculated. They were
quite punitive with me about this, even though I am not
afraid for Aaron to get the measles. I believe, as many re-
searchers do, that normal childhood illnesses build a
strong, natural immune system. And I'm convinced that the
immunities I passed from my own strong constitution into
Aaron's body through breast-feeding have already contributed to his good health.[9]

Whenever he has become ill or had difficulty, we always
attempt to feel into the problem, listen for guidance, and do
what is needed in the most natural, organic way in order to
help Aaron return to health. But on this particular night, I
temporarily lost my mind and ended up sitting in the emergency room of the hospital waiting for medical attention. I
called Aaron's daddy at work so he could meet us there.
Jonathan, who himself has a deeply instinctual and shamanic approach to healing, was appalled to hear we were
there and came as quickly as he could.

He sat down with Aaron in his arms and went into a
deep state of intentional meditation or trance, during which
Aaron "slept" for half an hour. Then, abruptly, Aaron woke

up, jumped down from his dad's lap, and began to run around the room, playing and laughing and asking to go home. We finally gave him his way. Having waited three hours, Aaron surely would have been acutely ill or dead if he had been poisoned or had appendicitis. We left the hospital with the nurses and the receptionist demanding that we wait to see the doctor, who they were certain would be with us very shortly. It seemed altogether ridiculous. I was incredibly sorry that I had come at all.

In retrospect, I was able to recall the odd events leading to his becoming sick. I remembered that he had seemed fine, and then when we walked up the steps, he had suddenly gasped and doubled over. It is possible that Aaron Eagle encountered a negative energy of some kind. If that was true, then what I should have done in that first moment was to burn sage to make it go away. Then if he had been poisoned or was having appendicitis, it would have become more obvious. Even with all my years of being a healer and treating my own illnesses in this way, as a mother I simply didn't function with my full range of instincts and intelligence. Under stress, I can still fall back into conditioned helplessness and powerlessness, wanting someone to rescue my child from danger. The emergency room event took on a humorous aspect for me when I was no longer worried about Aaron Eagle's health and I thought of him just getting up and running out of the hospital.

When Aaron first started public school, it did seem as though he got more colds and bronchial ailments. He would be out of school for a week, and I sneaked herbal remedies into his juice and got him to take homeopathic pills. Now that he has been in the school environment for several years, he is again strong and immune to most of the illnesses that the other children get. When he seems to be getting sick (if he gets listless, pale, tired, unaccountably unhappy or morose), I quickly give him a homeopathic remedy for colds and flu, which nips it in the bud. Once when I was in England for two weeks teaching, I woke up one morning from a dream in which Aaron was getting strep throat and I was worrying about him. My own throat itched when I woke up, and in my half-asleep state, I made a strong wish that I could somehow get the illness for him. I knew it seemed crazy, but I knew that I could heal myself as he would not be able to, and I was afraid nobody would be able to figure out what to do with him if he got something serious like strep throat while I was gone. Within several hours, I suddenly got sick with fever, headache, nausea, an overall tired feeling, and a very, very sore throat. My hostess drew a hot bath for me, made ginger tea, and sent me to bed. I sweated for six hours and slept through the rest of the night. I was well in the morning, and I called home to learn that Aaron had appeared to be coming down with a cold, but it went away the same day, and they had already sent him back to school.

Natural healing has an element of mystery that must always be allowed for. If we refer to it as magic, then people get nervous and think it is not real, that it's "superstitious," or a "work of the devil." But doesn't Western medicine seem equally superstitious, believing that illness is solely caused by aliens (germs) and that to heal it you have to kill them? Or that symptoms can be treated as isolated phenomena, separate from the whole body, the whole system? The body is an organism made up of many different complex systems — the glandular system, the organ system, the skeletal system, the muscular system. In the center of it all is the immune system, which is intricately related to brain messages and emotions, whereby if a person feels happy, she is likely to be healthy; if he feels depressed, he is likely to get sick.

I facilitate group ritual healing circles as part of my international teaching work. Wherever I go, people gather together, and in the context of drumming and chanting, we lay hands on those who are suffering from life-threatening illnesses in order to support their natural healing processes. In the course of my work, I have seen, after hands-on healing, a measurable rise in the T cell count of an AIDS patient and the blood count of a cancer patient; I have seen brain tumors shrink and disappear without any other treatment. Clients have reported back to me that their Pap smears came out normal following our work, and I have felt fibroid tumors shrink under my own hands.

I don't know why Aaron would get a fever for someone else's healing, or what would cause me to be able to take on his illness for him and heal it long-distance. But I know it's true, and I have learned to put my faith in that invisible process of healing that is always taking place in some other dimension of reality, right next to the one in which we live. In cultures that practices earth-based shamanism, these ideas would not seem peculiar at all. Anthropology has documented shamanic healing methods from all over the world, many of which are still practiced today right alongside Western techniques.

Shamans use dreams and visions, intuitions, feelings, and family interactions in their cures of individual illnesses. A child in a tribal culture is not isolated and expected to sleep alone in a hospital bed at night because she or he has become seriously ill. Tribal people don't hook up an IV and drip chemicals into the veins of a small child or keep it in an incubator because it's too small to be out on its own. A preemie in a tribal culture is wrapped warmly and kept close to the mother's breast until it reaches the correct (viable) weight, and the constant loving touch of its mother is what heals it. A sick child in a "primitive" culture would be put in the center of the tribal ceremony while the members of the community drum and dance (maybe for several days) until they have generated enough healing power to put their hands on the child and heal her. If there were "causes" that needed determining in order to rid the child of her illness, the whole family would be invited to participate in the ceremony, so that the whole system would be healed.

Aaron has always responded warmly to the use of rattles, drums, and hands-on healing for his own illnesses. He likes to be held and cuddled when he's sick, to be close to his loved ones and feel their grounded, loving touch; he naturally sleeps more than usual. If I am clear with him about the necessity, he will swallow the foulest-tasting herbal medicines now through his own volition. I share these stories about alternative approaches to Aaron's health because I believe the visible veil that hangs over so many children with Down syndrome, causing them to be lethargic and listless, can be lifted by a different approach to their health and healing. The rather constant illness that plagues so many of them can be eliminated with the right approach to their daily lives in terms of diet and activity, and this approach is known as "energy medicine."

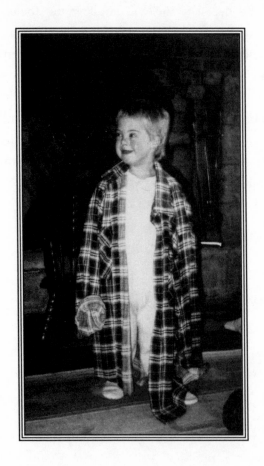

Aaron Eagle in big sister's flannel shirt,
age three. Photo by Jonathan Tenney.

Chapter Four

Wounded Healer

꒰

W HEN JONATHAN AND I LEARNED THAT AARON
had Down syndrome, we were momentarily shocked, and
our peace of mind was temporarily disrupted. But for some
parents, I know it's even worse; the initial revelation is un-
bearably difficult to handle, and it can take years to digest
and accept. One of the first essays we were given from
friends dealt with the never-ending grief of the parents of
handicapped children, a grief for the child you imagined that
never will be.[1] Over the years I have only very occasionally
come into contact with such feelings.

My first experience, as I have indicated, was more one of
wonder and receptivity. I had expected our child to be special; it just hadn't occurred to me he might be "handicapped."

At the time of Aaron's birth I was thirty-seven, and even with the doctor's office worrying over the ominous possibility of my giving birth to a child with Down syndrome, it had simply never entered my mind as something to fear. I had no preconceived notions about it and no set way to react. I wasn't interested in having amniocentesis in order to find out whether the baby I carried had an extra chromosome, because I wasn't going to terminate the pregnancy on account of that.

One of the things I've become aware of since Aaron's birth is how isolated disabled people are from the rest of us, and we from them. I had never had direct contact with "special" people until Aaron came to me. Disability is the stigma of being different writ large. Our society is so phobic of the "other" that anyone who is unusual or "not normal" is suspect and often persecuted. We may call ourselves the "melting pot," but we don't act like one. Without any firsthand experience of people with disabilities (or the "differently-abled," as they call themselves), how can we know how to receive them, how to act, talk, think, and interact with them? I see people struggling with this issue in regard to Aaron every day, and I feel sympathetic, because I myself felt the same confusion before he came into my life.

I'm not talking about the people who actually hate the handicapped and wish they had not been allowed to survive; they are a minority. Most people seem open but confused, uncertain of the "right" protocol in relation to a person with a physical or mental handicap. As a young teenager growing up in the Midwest, I was in a bowling league that met each Saturday morning. It was a lot of fun, and I have good memories from it. I like to think of the word *handicap* in the context of bowling, because there the higher handicap became a plus for our team, adding points to equalize things among all the participants. So you could be a great bowler, scoring over 200 a game, and be on a team with somebody who kept a 68 average. In that case, the teammate was given a certain number of points as a "handicap," which was added to your team's overall score. There is something comforting about this use of the word that has remained with me since we were informed of Aaron's condition.

Aaron is definitely a plus on our team. Although many of his skills are not at the same level as the rest of us, he is a delight to be around and adds something intangible, yet powerful, to our healthy functioning. Without him, we would be only normal. With him, we are expanded, stretched beyond who we knew ourselves to be. He's like a "contrary," in the Native American sense of the word, a sacred clown. The Sioux clown is called a *heyoka* and is "a man or woman who has received the greatest possible vision, that of the Thunder Being, who is many but only one, moves counter-sunwise instead of sunwise, is shapeless but has wings, lacks feet but has huge talons, and is headless but has a huge beak; his voice is the thunderclap and the glance of his eye is lightning."[2]

Like such a clown, Aaron Eagle is always throwing a curve into what would otherwise be the usual way of things.

One day recently, he put his shirt on his legs as pants, and vice versa, just as if he knew how a sacred clown should act! The ethnographer Barbara Tedlock describes how:

> During a heyoka impersonation, the new heyoka does many seemingly foolish things, such as riding backwards on his horse with his boots on backwards so that he's coming when he's really going; if the weather is hot he covers himself with blankets and shivers as with the cold, and he always says "yes" when he means "no." These actions . . . have important meaning. . . ."Fooling around, a clown is really performing a spiritual ceremony. . . ." The contrary actions of the heyoka not only demonstrate some of the unnatural, anti-sunwise nature of the Thunder Being, but they also open people.[3]

Aaron's innate sense of humor very much fits into Tedlock's description of the heyoka. He thinks it's absolutely hilarious when he can get people to do the opposite of what is expected or appropriate in any given situation. He is especially capable of getting our housemate, Karen Vogel, to act crazy with him and make contrary-like actions. He had a game he used to play of saying no when he meant yes, and vice versa, and then roaring with laughter.

Aaron keeps things creatively unstable, loose, with the unexpected always present. He lives very much in the moment, and he just doesn't do things the way other people do.

Contraries in the Cheyenne tradition do everything back-
wards and make everybody in the tribe laugh at their antics.
Tedlock says, "The clown's mystical liberation from ultimate
cosmic fears brings with it a liberation from conventional
notions of what is dangerous or sacred in the religious ceremonies of men [sic]." She goes on to theorize that the
clown, rather than weakening the social fabric, actually may
strengthen it, revitalizing it "by revealing higher truths."[4]
There is something very similar in the Tantric tradition in
India in the way that "crazy yogis" are perceived as living
outside the conventions that apply to normal citizens.[5]

In those first weeks after we were given Aaron Eagle's
"diagnosis," I felt challenged by the *heyoka* of this task suddenly facing me, this unknown destiny unfolding itself before my eyes. Jonathan and I felt like co-conspirators,
asking each other, "What will it mean?" It seemed, in a peculiar way, thrilling and sacred. The Goddess had seen fit
to give us something bigger than normal, something we
would have to rise to, that we could not take for granted. A
parent always wonders who this new child will be, what
form his or her unfolding will take. Every child is special
and has a destiny, and all children have the capacity to
open the hearts of their waiting parents on arrival.

But this child affected me differently from the beginning.
Thrown open, I found myself more present than usual,
awake to the subtle energies of the spirit world, which
seemed close enough to touch. The spirit energies seemed to
be coming into our house and into our life through the

channel of this odd little being who had come to be our child. I felt Aaron's spirit as quite large and somewhat imposing, perhaps bigger than my own. He seemed divine in some direct way, an elf or spirit-being himself. Part of this experience was no doubt just the sense of surprise and a result of being knocked off balance. But much of it was a real influx of subtle, invisible energy that comes through him still.

Tedlock believes that the "ability of American Indian religions to allow room for the disruptive, crazy, but creative power of the clown is perhaps their greatest strength." She says, "By startling people in these ways clowns reverse their polarity, as it were, curing them by releasing them from any idle thoughts or worries. This clearing of worry from the mind is both an ethical value and an important preventative health concept." She speaks of "the laughter that goes with a sudden opening or dislocation in the universe."[6] I can truly say that Aaron Eagle's unexpected and shocking arrival cleared my mind for quite a few years!

It helps parents of a child like Aaron Eagle to have some paradigms other than the pathological. Besides being "brain-injured" or "retarded," Aaron Eagle is brilliant, funny, open, surprising, and frequently transforms by just being present—truly a sacred Fool. A disabled person's life seems plagued by the rigid picture other people hold of his or her abilities. If he's "retarded," then naturally you wouldn't expect this little boy to be a genius at anything. "Differently-abled" people have gifts that go unnoticed by those around them, who fail to see what's there and see only what is missing. Like other people with Down syndrome, Aaron Eagle is amazing.

I don't mean to deny the difficulties or hardships in raising a special child like Aaron. It's inconvenient and labor-intensive to have a child in diapers for eight years; it takes enormous patience and an ongoing practice of loving-kindness to stay in right relation to his needs on a daily basis. Living with him is like having our personal Buddha in the house, forcing us to work on ourselves nonstop, with no slack. What's so bad about that? How else would we have the good sense to make changes, and the courage to carry through? That the rewards clearly outweigh the sacrifices is clear to anyone who has eyes to see.

On the second day of Aaron's life, as I was holding his little body and nursing him, someone put on the stereo a tape of meditative music that I had listened to throughout my pregnancy. I used to get in the bathtub at night and sink into deep relaxation, listening to this particular compilation of favorite songs that a friend had made for us. Tiny Aaron Eagle, only twenty-four hours old, began to push against my body in a deliberate rhythm, rocking himself in time to the beat of the music he had listened to for nine months. I was dumbfounded that such a thing was possible, but he was proving it by doing the impossible.

There is a magical aura surrounding Aaron that stops people in their tracks. I realized right away that one thing that would be difficult for me in raising Aaron would be other people's picture of him and the prevailing negative definition of his "condition." I remember a time when Aaron was a tiny boy sitting in the front of my grocery cart while we waited in a checkout line behind a very irritated woman. She suddenly turned, noticed him without really seeing him, and began to interact right in his face in a nervous, unconscious way. "Hi there," she said, kind of poking him with her finger. He squinched up his face, frowned, stuck out his jaw, and made the most awful noise at her, like a wild animal. She jumped back and left him alone after that, while I tried to act "normal." Ho hum. Nothing unusual here, just my little guy reflecting reality back at you like a Buddhist mirror.

"What's wrong with him, Mommy?" ask some children who recoil from his appearance or his behavior, and in spite of what I know, I feel hurt for him and me. Like other children with Down syndrome, Aaron's tongue sometimes hangs out of his mouth, he drools, he moves his body in an awkward way, or his words come out funny. I have to keep myself from trying to fix him. His appearance and his behavior change dramatically according to how he feels and the state of his health. He is so transparent that whatever is happening around him is likely to leave its mark on him.

We have been forced to raise our vibrations around Aaron, for his sake. The clear mirror he presents is a direct spiritual teaching, and we find ourselves necessarily changing for the better. There were ways that Jonathan and I transformed in the first year of Aaron's life that have contributed enormously to the character of each of us. I was a screamer all my life—nobody has ever been able to get me to stop when I felt justifiably angry about something. My relationship with Jonathan was quite intense and passionate, leading to a good deal of open fighting over the years that had become rather habitual by the time Aaron Eagle was with us.

One day, Aaron was sitting on my knee in the living room of our Arizona house, and Jonathan and I got into a fight. I began to yell at him, outraged, infuriated, out of control. And then I looked at the face of the little person sitting on my lap, wide-eyed, mouth agape. I was shocked to watch Aaron become "retarded" right in front of me, in a matter of moments. The negative energy was simply too strong for him, and he couldn't process it; he disintegrated. It's not as though he thought about it, or cried, or got visibly upset. He just became ill, absorbing the toxins, as if a terrible veil came down over him. It was a profound, inarguable teaching, flooding me with shame. I promised I would never scream like that again.

Jonathan, on the other hand, never knew how to express his anger and would go into a cold, detached, separated space for days at a time when he was mad. Before Aaron was born, I had tried to get Jonathan to change, just as he had tried to get me to stop screaming, but to no avail. Aaron could not handle the cold isolation of his daddy's depressions and would become heavy and lethargic. In no time at all, Jonathan realized for himself that he could not continue to allow these dark moods to take over because it was so hard on Aaron Eagle. Like me, he had to get control over himself. By the end of Aaron's first year with us, he had accomplished what no parent, friend, or partner had been able to achieve: the permanent transformation of our evil ways. What clearer sign of holiness is there in any person than that he or she has the power to effect transformation in other people?

In a tribal culture, where magic is revered and the unseen is understood to be sacred, a child like Aaron Eagle might be recognized as a shaman or a sacred clown. He has the gift of reaching out and touching, making contact with others, and raising their spirits through this interaction. It's as if he came into the world with this as his task, or "dharma," as the Buddhists say. He has the kind of equilibrium glorified in spiritual disciplines, in which he relates to everyone the same way, with no hierarchy and few preferences.

When we first moved from Arizona back to Berkeley, we would go out for walks, and Aaron would always approach the "street people" sitting on benches or in doorways. He was never put off by their rough appearance or the fact that they might be high on something, or depressed, or hurting. In fact, it was to this hurt that he seemed drawn. The most isolated cases seemed to attract his focused attention, and he would approach the lonely, desperate people with his hand out, saying, "Hey!" to get their attention, to pull them out of themselves long enough to brighten their day.

When he was about six months old, Aaron discovered himself in a mirror. He was transfixed and has stayed that way. He talks to himself, gestures, tells stories, imitates things he has seen others do, sings, shows off, tries on hats and various expressions. In short, he has the kind of healthy, loving relationship with himself that every one of us needs and most of us don't know how to get. He seems to think he's great, yet he doesn't push that onto others as an aggression. His self-esteem is neutral and innate. His natural detachment and curiosity serve him well in the area of performance and musical theater as well. He has no self-consciousness and therefore can try on anything for size.

Aaron is always happiest as the center of attention, whether he's performing for himself in the mirror or for hundreds of people at a public event. When put in front of a microphone and given permission to use it, Aaron is blissfully content. He can go on and on, playing his harmonica, talking to the people, laughing, singing, taking a bow. Given a chance, he would lead any program himself. Because my work involves public speaking and group ceremonies, Aaron has had ample opportunities over the years to express himself in this way. I have always been impressed at the level of sophistication he manifests in these public arenas. He has no fear of crowds, and he has the ability to channel high-voltage energies usually reserved for preachers and performing artists. He responds naturally to the rhythm of the crowd.

Shortly after we moved back to the Bay Area, I produced a large ritual event in San Francisco at the Galleria Design Center, a four-story renovated warehouse that has become an elegant indoor, skylit garden theater. Nine hundred

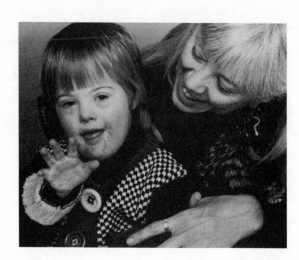

Vicki and
Aaron
Eagle,
age four.
Photo by
Irene
Young.

participants came for the day to do ritual, see dance and musical presentations, and hear speakers like Riane Eisler and Daniel Patricia Ellsberg on the subject of healing the earth. The day culminated with Motherpeace co-creator Karen Vogel leading a spiral dance up, down, and around all four stories, to the rhythmic sounds of the Sons of Orpheus, a local men's drumming group. In the morning, I gave a keynote talk on the state of the world, with Aaron Eagle as the central subject.

The talk had come to me in a magical way, unlike any previous public lecture I had given. I was sitting in the kitchen one day with little Aaron pushing a truck back and forth on the tile floor nearby. It was very peaceful, and I was enjoying his quiet company. Suddenly I felt as if something came into me, pushing me into an altered state of consciousness in which I began to hear the speech inside my head, as if it were an essay already written. I got paper and pen and began to write it as I was hearing it. When I was near the end of the piece, musing on its purpose, I suddenly knew it was the talk I would deliver at the earth-healing event that was still six weeks away. Up until that moment, I had planned to speak at the event about feminism and women healing the planet.

Instead, I spoke directly to the audience from the paper I had written that day in my kitchen, all about living with little Aaron Eagle and what that had to do with the state of the world. I had never read a speech from a text before, as I always tend to improvise in the moment in my public speaking. As I spoke that day, it became absolutely still in the room, and people seemed to drop to a deeper level of consciousness within the first few paragraphs. I understood that there was something universal about Aaron Eagle, and that the points I wished to make to people that day could best be made through his story.

After my talk, which lasted only about twenty minutes, Aaron's daddy released him from behind the curtains and he came running out on stage and into my arms. He was fascinated by the hundreds and hundreds of people in the audience, and not at all afraid, so I let him speak into the microphone for a moment. When I put him down again, the morning part of the program was officially ended, and we were leading into a lunch break. In the ensuing chaos, I lost track of him. He had gotten down from the stage and gone out into the circle of people in front, where he began shaking hands. People described it to me later: Aaron Eagle greeting each person individually, almost as if he was saying, "Welcome to my Mom and Dad's living room, nice to have you," as he shook eighty hands in turn. It was an extremely poignant moment for many people whose lives he touched that day.

A shaman is a wounded healer, and Aaron embodies this archetype. He came into this life with a visible handicap, and he heals everyone he comes into contact with through his simplicity, his genuineness, and his charismatic power. Through rising above his own disability every day, Aaron models for humanity the possibilities implicit in each of us, no matter how damaged we might be. Since so many of us feel ourselves to be damaged in invisible ways, this healing act on his part is profound for us. Although severely limited in some dimensions of his existence, Aaron is highly evolved in others. He has an awesome stage presence, and his stage is the world.

For several years now, Karen Vogel has lived in the same house with Aaron and me. (For some of those years, Jonathan and his mother, Marga, lived here as well.) A few years ago, when Aaron was about four years old, Karen was studying conga drumming with a local teacher, Carolyn Brandy, and they were having their drumming class in our living room. Aaron was invited to join the group for a while, and he spontaneously locked into a rhythm with Carolyn, who was playing a wild solo to the group's steady beat. Aaron became carried away with the totality of the thing and was able to "entrain" with her through his body, not his mind. It looked like a big chill went through his body for a moment, and he undulated with it. It was one of those amazing moments in music, when everybody gets in the "groove" and there is a complete unity.

Joachim-Ernst Berendt, author of *Nada Brahma: The World Is Sound*, explains entrainment as "the tendency of everything that vibrates—in other words, everything—to swing together, to lock in . . . the tendency of the universe to share rhythms, to vibrate in harmony." He says entrainment is universal in nature and is a physical phenomenon that can be witnessed in animal behavior. Groups of birds or fish, for instance, who function as a single organism when they are migrating or swimming in a school, never collide, yet follow no set leader. The command, Berendt says, comes from the group as a whole and not from a single animal as science had first assumed. He goes on to describe disease as "the formation of chaotic rhythms" and cancer as "rhythmic chaos" in which there is a total irregularity of all rhythms because the cancer cell "withdraws from the temporal harmony of the body functions." He quotes the poet Novalis: "Every disease is a musical problem."[7]

Aaron Eagle heals disease in people and in society, not because he has a strong rational mind and knows linear techniques, but because he is able to give himself up to the music. According to esoteric spiritual teachings, the whole universe was created from sound, and is sound. As Berendt points out, there is a rushing stream, a river of sound (*nadi*) that is the underlying structure of everything. And it is not chaotic or random, but tends toward harmony. "All dissonances," Berendt contends, "gravitate toward becoming harmonies."[8] Aaron Eagle is an intuitive, open channel for such a movement toward unification and well-being. He lacks the kind of ego-control that drives the rest of us and keeps us from letting go into the flow. Aaron is a specialist in the art of surrender, the state of "being here now." He especially likes folk music and rock 'n' roll, but I think he's hearing the true sounds behind everything—the "Nada Brahma."

A friend gave me a tape of music written and performed by the Navajo singer Sharon Burch in her native tongue. The songs are traditional chants set to contemporary melodies, and her voice is strong and beautiful. Aaron heard the tape and sang along as if he knew the language; it was eerie. He couldn't talk, but he seemed to know songs in Navajo, and for years he requested that we play the tape whenever we got in the car. There was one special song called "The Chant" that he made me play again and again.[9]

Our close family friend Jennifer Berezan is also a singer, songwriter, and performer. Aaron and I often accompany her to local events. Aaron knows all Jennifer's songs by heart, because, in addition to her performances, he insists on listening to her two tapes when we drive. We listen not once, not twice, but over and over, sometimes all the way to Santa Cruz to visit Aaron's big sisters (a ninety-minute drive), with Aaron singing at the top of his lungs, shaking a rattle, and playing harmonica along with the music.

In any circle of children at school, camp, festivals, and so on, Aaron is the center of attention, performing a song or dance freely, uninhibited by the ego-fixations, doubts, or fears of normal people. His utter lack of self-consciousness makes music an arena of leadership and self-expression for him with his peers. It gives him opportunities that would not otherwise exist for him, because when people are making music, the rules of the social scene suddenly make sense to him. His enjoyment is unbounded, and he will try anything! He doesn't stand outside himself or wonder how he looks; he simply allows the music or rhythm to inform him in the body, and he expresses that. For this reason, we believe Aaron was born to perform.

Aaron's harmonica playing has become legendary. He plays the instrument with feeling. He will perform anytime, anywhere, on stage or off, for the family or for hundreds of strangers. He can make it have vibrato by changing the position of his hands, and he has a bluesy approach to holding the notes on long in-and-out breaths. It's as if he has an innate skill at something that he can't understand or learn in a conceptual way at all yet. In a public event in Berkeley sponsored by Gaia bookstore, owner Patrice Wynne introduced Aaron Eagle as the special guest who would "open the ritual for us tonight." Aaron came to the microphone like a professional, spoke a few measured words to the audience, and then began to blow his mouth organ in rhythm to the beat of the crowd. He was, as he always is, extremely pleased with himself and life, and he happily accepted the applause from the crowd.

Once Jennifer finished a concert and left the stage, while people stamped and clapped and shouted for an encore. Swept up in the excitement of the moment, Aaron, who was sitting with me in the front row, jumped up and faced the audience with his arms outstretched, accepting the adulation for himself and channeling the currents of energy through his own body. Jennifer came back onstage and generously asked him to say a few words and take a bow, which he was happy to do, and which the audience reinforced with their praise.

In these public moments, which are becoming more common in Aaron's life, he is equally without ego and without embarrassment, absolutely in the moment and flowing with the energy. Creation speaks through this boy, sings through him, moves through him, and by his uninhibited expression he touches others with that mysterious ecstatic joy that belongs to the realm of divinity. This expression is not personal for Aaron, but simply life pulsating through him in a song. He cannot help himself, he has to sing, he has to dance, and he does it for you and me. His performances are actual transformations of the energies in the room and in the people. Clearly a healer, he changes consciousness by his openness, his freshness. His singing and dancing seem to have a deeper, more magical purpose than simply to entertain.

What a shame it would be if we saw Aaron only through the filter of Down syndrome! What if the people in his life assumed he couldn't achieve anything out of the ordinary, in fact, could not even come up to what we call normal? What if it were a decade earlier and we had given Aaron up to be institutionalized, on the advice of his doctor, because he might be a "burden" to us, to his family or society? Or what if we merely sat him in front of a TV and never had any expectations of his greatness?

It's not that Jonathan and I attach to specific goals in relation to Aaron. We don't assume he must do anything in particular, until he shows a tendency in that direction. And we never assume there is anything he won't be able to do if he wants to. (Will he read? Will he write? Who knows, who cares? Let him show us what he came here to do.) After he demonstrates some leaning toward an activity or skill, we try to nurture its development in him by providing him with opportunities: materials or teachers or whatever context will make the thing grow. We watch to see what seeds come up, and then we water them. Period. We take advantage of the artists and musicians who have come into his life, the special teachers and tutors who reach out to him, as well as his older sisters and their loved ones.

Not long ago, while I was driving the car and Aaron was singing in the backseat, I realized that for the first time he was singing something familiar, the melody of which I could recognize ("Jingle Bells"), and that in that moment, we had crossed another milestone in his development. He has always *heard* the melody in a song, but now he is beginning to be able to *reproduce* it. This will be life-changing for any destiny he might have as a performer. Mary Mackey, a friend of mine who writes novels, once pointed out to me the important difference between expression and communication. Expression, she said, exists for itself, and I think of Aaron's precious babbling that no one understands besides himself. Communication, on the other hand, is when you make an expression that someone else understands and can receive. Aaron, like many people with Down syndrome, is just dying to communicate.

He has always had a distinct social sense and an uncanny ability to intuit what is needed in mundane group situations. I've seen Aaron sense the underlying tensions between me and his dad, for example, and then insist that we give each other a hug before going on to any other business. I've watched him press for strangers to meet each other and shake hands, or even hug. He took my mother to school one day when she was visiting from Iowa, and he introduced her to each of the teachers in his special education room one at a time, by name, and insisted that they all shake hands and say hello. At parties in our community, he seems to be attracted to the single individual sitting uncomfortably alone, or to a young person who needs contact, or to someone who would not normally open up to conversation with a stranger. He can break down the barriers and open hearts, and he seems to have a fairly good sense of when to loosen up normally formal situations.

He has recently taken up being a waiter. Having watched so many waiters and waitresses over the years, he suddenly decided he wanted to be the waiter himself. He got up from the table recently in a fancy restaurant when we had finished our meal and began conversing with the woman at the next table. Before I knew it, she had pulled out a small tablet and pencil from her purse and given it to Aaron Eagle, who was standing at attention, ready to take her order. Without his being able to tell her in words exactly what he had in mind, his body language had been so clear that she was reading things off the menu and telling him what she wanted as he wrote the imaginary items down on his tablet. He was nodding and gesturing, saying, "Yes, yes, okay," and writing things down. Then, when he was finished, he set off to other tables to do the same thing. I attempted to stop him, thinking that he was bothering people, but all the people at the neighboring tables overruled me by encouraging him. I had difficulty getting him out of there that night, so eager was he to take everyone's order and serve them their pretend food!

It may be superstitious of me, but I believe Aaron Eagle chose me and his dad, not for a linear, disciplined approach, but because we are healers and artists and, no matter what else, we live the creative life. Aaron Eagle is just bursting with creativity, which seems to want to take the strongest, most enduring form through music and theater. I've seen him on stage bringing joy and transformation to all kinds of people through his loving, open heart. He is currently painting, playing golf, and playing his new drum set. He's very good at mime and clowning. He knows all the lines of the *Wee Sing* videos (no small task), and lately he has shown an intense interest in martial arts. We can hardly keep up with him when he gets into one of his frequent growth spurts.

Limit his choices? Not a chance. For Aaron Eagle, the sky's the limit.

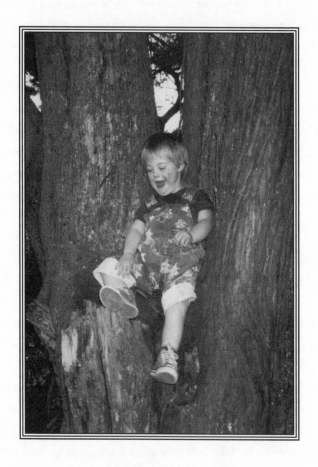

Aaron Eagle in tree, age six.
Photo by Jonathan Tenney.

Chapter Five

In His Own Time

ॐ

DELAYS IN LEARNING CREATE A KIND OF TIME warp in the developmental period of a child's life. When Aaron was first born, he didn't cry. For weeks (perhaps months) he didn't smile. I remember his first smile. He and I were out walking on the road near our desert home in Arizona, with him bundled in a carrier against my chest. As I walked, I looked down at his little face and became aware of my own sad feelings that he wasn't able to return my smile. Other babies smiled long before this, of course, and I suddenly felt that I couldn't stand waiting any longer. I felt how much I wanted this baby to smile, how I wanted to encounter him personally through his ability to express himself like that.

And just as simply as that, he looked up at me and flashed me his first gentle, but definite, smile. I nearly fell over. After that, he knew how to do it, and he has been quite a happy, smiling boy since!

Waiting plays a central role for parents of special children. The waiting literally never ends. I have found it necessary to think of it as a spiritual practice, like meditation—concentrating on a long-term evolutionary goal without becoming invested in the actual outcome. We have to put our minds on the goal in a gentle, "allowing" kind of way, without grasping, without attachment. Usually we go through a period of wanting the thing to happen ("It must be time for Aaron to sit up"), getting impatient after several weeks or months without success ("He just doesn't seem to get it"), and finally practically giving up ("Oh well, maybe he never will sit up"). Then one ordinary day like any other, and without any apparent reason, he manages to sit himself up and stay in that position. He enjoys it, he learns to do it routinely, and before too long we hardly remember what it was like before he couldn't sit up.

But then it's time for him to crawl. He wants to. He tries. He gets himself up on all four legs, makes an effort to move forward, crashes down on his belly, and seems to feel frustrated over the failed attempt. Is it possible he's conscious of his own condition? It seems as though he's afraid to try after a failure. This goes on for months, until one day (many, many months later) it clicks, and he's crawling for the next year or two without a problem. Except that by then, we're wanting him to walk, and we're helping him to try, and we're hoping . . . and praying . . . and, as always, waiting.

Aaron finally took his first step in the wide open, carpeted field of the airport in Salt Lake City, where he and I had a layover on our way to visit my family in the Midwest. There we were, trapped with hundreds of other traveling folks, waiting our turn to get on the next plane, and Aaron just up and walked across the room. He fell on his face, laughed, got up, walked some more, fell again, and repeated the whole thing in front of total strangers for two hours. It was as though he was using the time to practice. The big event we had all been waiting for for over a year (he was two and a half) took place in one instant in a public arena away from home—away from his daddy, his sisters, his aunties, and all the supportive people at preschool who wished to see him accomplish this important milestone.

"How old is he?" asks a stranger in an outdoor restaurant in Berkeley. Aaron and I are sitting in the sunshine, eating frozen yogurt—one of his favorite activities—and the woman has come over to sell us something.

"Six," I answer, knowing that she is searching for something to explain him.

"He's unusual," she suggests.

"He's a special boy," I agree, "he has Down syndrome."

"What does that mean?"

"It means he has an extra chromosome, his learning is delayed, and his heart is wide open," I answer, trying to sum up Aaron Eagle in one cryptic sentence.

She, like so many people who encounter Aaron, is visibly moved by him, and by my description of him. Aaron proceeds to grin at her, lick his chocolaty lips, and string a long series of syllables together in response to her attention.

How old is he? has become a commonplace question in our lives, as people attempt to make sense out of what they are seeing. Aaron Eagle is the same size or slightly smaller than other children his age, with a bright personality that includes wanting to interact with strangers. People often assume when Aaron speaks to them that they should be able to understand him, and they cannot. They look questioningly at me, but I often don't know the answer either. Over the years his articulation and his body movements get clearer, but still he is always noticeably different. Usually this difference is perceived as Aaron's being younger than he is.

Americans are fast. We like to do things in a hurry, accomplish a lot in a little time, and basically get the job done and get on with it. Everybody I know is moving at a pretty fast clip, from this activity to that one, and we believe the reward is the achievement of the goal in as little time as possible. Now meditation teachers have been bringing us a message about another approach to life, and some of us have attempted to slow ourselves down enough to at least include a little relaxation in our otherwise busy schedules. But Aaron's pace is a total confrontation to "normal" ways of moving in the world. Aaron's development (his accomplishment of tasks) is so slow, it is downright un-American.

As in the old tale of the tortoise and the hare, Aaron moves through the normal milestones of childhood like an even-tempered turtle who gets to the finish line when he gets there. The rest of us are in a totally different time scale, and it takes extraordinary patience (and self-development in ourselves) to wait with good humor and nurture his incremental steps toward success. All parents of children with learning disorders or disabilities know what I'm talking about. It is painstakingly laborious to facilitate Aaron's learning without projecting on him that he's a problem. And because it takes a cheerful and steady approach to motivate him to even try certain tasks, impatience is an absolutely unacceptable way of relating to him. Like the audience watching the Special Olympics, we must cheer Aaron on in every race he enters.

In simple physical terms, this means a labor-intensive upbringing. For example, although Aaron didn't walk until he was two-and-a-half, he weighed as much as any other child that age, and he had to be carried. That means a parent or caretaker had to carry him everywhere that he couldn't crawl by himself, and he was heavy! We all got stronger over time. I remember walking home from the corner market one day, having picked up a few items, which I was carrying in a grocery sack. Aaron had learned to walk, but he tired easily, and on this particular day, he simply couldn't make the walk home by himself. I had to carry him in one arm and the groceries in the other. It was a feat of will. I imagined that I was a Guatemalan peasant woman walking home from the market with a child and a bundle, and I knew I could do it if she could!

I developed Amazon fantasies, and stamina to match. I carried Aaron at age two in a frame backpack, with all our travel needs in three separate carryons, all the way across O'Hare Airport in time to change planes to Iowa. I have a very funny snapshot of myself carrying him home to our house in Berkeley by the straps of his overalls, when he refused to cooperate with me by walking. There he is, dangling from my right arm, crying in frustration at me, while in my left arm is a large package from town. I am marching like a soldier, with a slight grin on my face.

Many so-called mentally retarded children have difficulty speaking in a way that can be understood, and this has been true for Aaron Eagle. During the early years, this lack of communication between Aaron and others was a source of continuous pain and struggle. He had so much to say, yet his words didn't come out the way he intended, and this disappointed and frustrated him to the point where he sometimes refused to try. In our culture, we depend very much on words and the exchange of ideas. Without words, it seems as if we don't understand one another deeply. There are times when I feel an unfathomable loss because I can't sit down and really read a story with Aaron or really have a conversation about how his day at school was. I long for that level of relationship with him. I know eventually it will come, but the waiting is intensely difficult.

I have a hot tub in my backyard, and I like to get in the tub at least once every day. Sometimes Aaron Eagle gets in with me, and we have a lovely time together. He might splash and "swim" and generally carry on, but there are moments of quiet that open up between us in this context.

One day about sunset, we got out of the tub and instead of going right in the house, we wrapped our towels around us and sat down together on the back stoop. I said to Aaron, "Sometimes after I take a hot tub, I like to sit here and listen to the sounds of the wind and the birds." He opened his senses and leaned his head on my shoulder, and I knew he totally understood what I was saying. It was one of those precious moments when we communicate as deeply as I could want with anyone.

Sometimes his lack of ability in talking, and our lack of ability to hear or understand him clearly, is frustrating and depresses him as well as the rest of us. When you can tell that your child has something specific he wants or needs, and he tries and tries to make you understand what it is, then gives up in hopelessness, it makes you feel bad, to say the least. Aaron, like many other "retarded" children, has his own special language, made up of strings of sounds and syllables rattled off quickly with all the complex and varied intonation that make up the sentences you and I use in speaking to each other. We have very much enjoyed his special language and the charming way he "talks" to and interacts with people. But we can't help but miss the nitty-gritty exchange of having him tell us, in understandable words, what he wants and how he wants it.

Think of when you first heard a toddler—less than two years old—say a whole sentence clearly. I remember my oldest daughter Robyn, when she was fourteen months old, looking out the car window in Portsmouth, New Hampshire, where we lived, and saying as clear as a bell, "Nook at the boat!" It was thrilling. Speech came easily and abundantly, and she was reading sentences by the age of three. She was a normal, and quite precocious, little girl.

When Aaron was small, we began to see that he could understand what was said to him, although he could not reproduce the sounds himself. I took heart in this fact, and began to invent ways of relating to him, guessing that he could understand me even though I couldn't prove it. Because he often doesn't think the same way we do, and because he can't talk in concepts and sentences, it is tempting to treat him as if he doesn't understand things that are actually within his grasp on a level other than the rational. I have to remind myself not to give up and to make the necessary effort to include him in our decisions and the events of our lives. When he is included, he doesn't feel the need to act out in order to get the attention he's missing, and the rest of us feel more connected and loved by him as well.

Sign language is a wonderful bridge between disabled persons and their world, but unfortunately most of us don't speak it. In Aaron's first preschool, the special education teacher used sign language with all the differently-abled kids, and Aaron thrived on it. He learned to ask for certain of his favorite foods by signing (crackers, juice, water, more), and for the first time we were able to respond to his desires directly. Then in the first years of elementary school, his teachers used sign very little, if at all, and Jonathan and I forgot most of what we had understood when Aaron was younger.

Sometimes the trouble is deeper than words or signing can deal with, and then the methods must be even more intuitive and nonrational. In many ways, Aaron has been transforming me over the years by simply being unable to do things my way. I have to either give up on him or open to the different ways he can do things, and the different things he can do. I think we are so unused to extending ourselves beyond the use of speech, and so frightened by anything out of the ordinary, that we shrink from encounters with differently-abled people and inflict on them more suffering than they already feel in relation to their own difficulties. If he were in a wheelchair, I couldn't be impatient with him for not jogging with me. We would simply have to find another way of being physical together, and chances are, it would best unfold if I could allow Aaron to show me what might be possible, rather than the other way around.

Since Aaron cannot keep up with us—he can't play most of our games, do our jobs, read our books, think our thoughts—we have had to slow down to a speed that can accommodate him. If we can't do that, the world passes him by very quickly, and he tends to give up trying to interact with it. He spaces out, making repetitive verbal sounds and drooling, and his eyes glaze over. The magic of the situation comes when we are able to align with him enough that we begin to reap the benefits of the slower speed. Very creative and funny ideas pop into being when Aaron is the director of the activity, and at times, the mystical opens through his lead.

Fifteen years ago, I often went to a Tibetan Buddhist center in Berkeley for dinner on Sunday nights. Thirty of us, strangers, would eat dinner in silence, using mindfulness practices while chewing our food instead of distracting ourselves from the activity of eating, in the usual way, by talking. It was a bit awkward, as such meditations always are for Westerners but interesting because it caused subtle changes to happen within. Now I eat a lot of my dinners alone with Aaron, who tends to eat silently and meditatively, just like a Buddhist.

Aaron has always tremendously enjoyed eating. His appetite is great, and he loves food. He seems to relate to his food with one-pointedness, giving it his full attention, in a way that the rest of us are not accustomed to doing. This is not to say that he doesn't also enjoy lively dinner conversation, because when other people join us for dinner, he is always very happy and excited about that. He becomes the life of the party, talking and joking and generally making everyone at the table laugh with pleasure at his entertainment. He loves a party. But during our peaceful, solitary mealtimes, he is quiet and contemplative. It is unbelievably spacious for me when this happens.

The same has been true of going walking with Aaron. Over the years, we have taken walks all over Berkeley and Oakland, up and down College Avenue to visit his favorite haunts: the yogurt shop, the used toy store, the mailboxes. I have spent many a Saturday in this leisurely way, letting little Aaron be the guide for our journeys, following him at his pace where he chose to go. I started this practice because when I tried to take him on my trip at my pace, he balked and made it very difficult for me. Much of the time when we were walking in his way (sometimes literally for hours at a time), we would not speak to each other but would simply be with each other, together, quietly. I am normally so extroverted in my life that this unintentional (on my part) nonverbal activity was at first uncomfortable, but later it became a welcome meditation for me. I began to experience my private time with Aaron as nourishing and relaxing in a way I had not anticipated.

When you are with a person without talking for long periods of time, some other form of communication begins to open. The senses shift their attention from the left-brain, rational mode, to a right-brain, intuitive, receptive way of being. The whole world looks and feels different in such a mode of perception. Tribal people, and people who love the quiet of nature, know about this way of being. Some artists know it, from their necessarily long periods of quiet painting or drawing or sculpting. Meditators know it. Breast-feeding mothers certainly know it.

I remember sitting in the rocking chair with Aaron as a baby, feeding and feeding him. It seemed as if whole days went by that way, with ideas and thoughts arising and disappearing without any action in their behalf. I would momentarily think that I wanted to say or do something, but since I was otherwise occupied, the thought or impulse would simply pass into oblivion, and I would continue the nursing. Buddhists call this "milk mind," but with Aaron Eagle this state is accessible more of the time. I am deeply grateful to him for showing me how to slow down enough to experience and appreciate the finer things in life.

There is nothing more challenging to wait for than toilet training. I can still hear Aaron's first preschool teacher, a specialist in Down syndrome, with her own child with Down syndrome as well, telling us with a kind of Buddhist compassion that her child did not potty-train until he was eight years old. I made a mental note that this would not be the case for us, that certainly through our unqualified attention and goodwill, Aaron would succeed at this basic bodily task much earlier than that. I really thought we wouldn't be able to stand it if he took that long; I simply couldn't imagine it. Now, Aaron Eagle is eight years old, and we have a team of intelligent adults almost totally focused on getting him to use the toilet regularly. And still, his successful and consistent potty-training has eluded us.

I can tell from experience in these matters that our progress on this one is near the completion point. But that could mean another year. I am betting that by the time this book is in print, Aaron will have gained access to the world of bowel and bladder control that the rest of us take for granted. But at the moment, it is still hit-and-miss. Sometimes he does, and just as often he doesn't. We work on this issue from morning until night, at school and out in the world and at Mommy's and Daddy's houses. Every caretaker and helper is made an aware part of the team dedicated to getting Aaron Eagle out of diapers. We wonder constantly, does he comprehend what we want in this matter? Is he willfully resisting us? If so, can we get around it?

One clue came the first time Aaron successfully initiated going to the toilet on his own. He was in a public place (a movie theater) with the babysitter who is his most playful, least discipline-oriented helper, the one person of the whole team least inclined to focus on Aaron's potty-training. She went to use the toilet herself, and when she came out of the stall, he had disappeared. Of course, she panicked at the thought of Aaron lost out in the world, and she looked everywhere for him. He turned out to be in the next stall, having taken off his own diaper and successfully used the toilet. After this, we were able to understand that in some very deep and primal way, Aaron wanted to be independent in this activity. He did not respond well to pressure.

Now his whole teaching team is shifting toward letting him be more self-directing in his use of the toilet. The teachers and aides who work with Aaron at public school, where he is integrated into a normal first-grade class, seized on the idea with relish. They don't take him to the bathroom anymore; they send him. And the most recent (and even more successful) intervention is that they send him with a little friend of his from first grade, a boy who has volunteered to take Aaron by the hand and accompany him to the bathroom in order for both of them to use it in a routine way. Aaron wears training pants to school, and all the aides and teachers who work with him in the course of the day are briefed as to the agreed-upon routine, so that his toileting can function at the highest possible level. Consistency and focused attention are the secrets. If there weren't this kind of order and cooperation on the part of the school staff and Aaron's child care workers, I doubt the project could succeed.

Because the learning is so slow and well defined in the case of someone with Down syndrome, there is an opportunity to see the details in the learning process itself. It is quite interesting to see how linear and step-by-step it is and yet how Aaron Eagle (and each of us, I imagine) spirals around and around in the process of moving ahead. There are no straight lines, and Aaron Eagle is here to prove it.

Sometimes the process of getting Aaron off to school in the morning is fraught with anxiety, because he moves so slowly, and I'm trying not to be late. I can wake up two or three hours before school time and still not get him there until after his class has started. It's not that he can't do what is needed; it is more that he won't. He resists. He just won't move. Sometimes he smiles mischievously at me. He knows I want him to get dressed, eat breakfast, and go to school. He actually likes school. But he just can't seem to entirely cooperate, so we have to trick, humor, coax, and tease him into compliance. A hand puppet of Ernie from "Sesame Street" has recently been very helpful. Games always help. Constant creativity is an absolutely necessary ingredient in our life together.

I have no choice but to think of being with Aaron Eagle as a spiritual practice, and clearly it is as effective as any other at helping with my personal evolution. Sitting on a pillow and staring at a blank wall, I could not cultivate any more patience or compassion than that which naturally comes to me when my heart is open to this little boy as he takes his sweet time getting where he's intended to go.

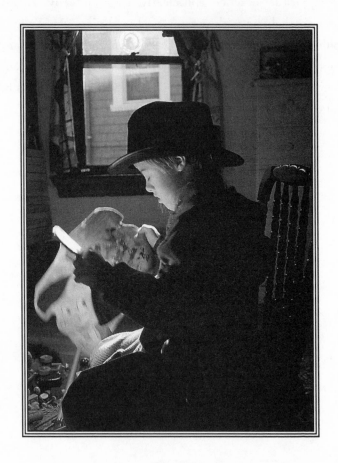

Aaron Eagle reading his favorite book, *Pinocchio*,
age six. Photo by Karen Vogel.

Chapter Six

Never Too
Much Stimulation

جرح

THERE ARE PROBABLY AS MANY DIFFERENT approaches to Down syndrome as there are parents of these special children. There is agreement across the board on the need for as much stimulation as early as possible. If the child with Down syndrome can be awakened and his or her energies significantly aroused before the age of five, then minor miracles can happen. There are "early infant stim" programs all over the world, developed for the purpose of pushing the "retarded" child past the old negative pictures of being untrainable. Rather than giving up on a developmentally disabled child, the idea is that parents can push for whatever might be possible within each child's particular destiny. The range of potential varies a great deal among children with Down syndrome and other chromosomal disorders, and nobody really knows what the limits are. Children with Down syndrome are now reading and writing, playing sports, and even becoming actors on television.

When Aaron was born, we received a copy of *Son-Rise*, a book by Barry Neil Kaufman about his son with autism and the heroic battle of the child's mother on her son's behalf. Through almost superhuman efforts Sue Kaufman was able to push her autistic child past all set limits applied to autism. The parents had to push to get the proper diagnosis and treatment for their child at an early age, and then after receiving the medical establishment's diagnosis of autism and their recommendation that the parents give up on such a hopeless child, the parents (especially the mother) worked eight hours or more a day to physically and actively stimulate the child into awareness and human contact. Miraculously, in the face of no significant response at first, the mother's unceasing efforts eventually paid off, and the child eventually progressed in amazing and unexpected ways. *Son-Rise* is a testimony to the parents' blind and instinctual faith in their child and the tireless application of this faith into real physical programming.

During Aaron's first few months, his unnatural quietude was a cause for our concern. It seemed as if he was in a kind of light slumber, or that he in some way had chosen to not yet fully incarnate. He was beyond placid. There seemed to be a bubble surrounding him, cutting him off from us and us from him. He didn't seem unhappy, just somehow lost to us, out of reach. He had a very special, almost angelic quality, but we wanted contact with him as a human being. In those first weeks, we read about the early learning "patterning" process utilized by Glenn Doman at the Institutes for the Achievement of Human Potential in Philadelphia. In their radical approach to mental retardation—that the brain itself must be treated, rather than the peripheral symptoms—the Institutes get their children to crawl and do other precise physical patterning activities over and over again—hundreds, even thousands of times, over a period of weeks or months or years. The children are put on a regimented schedule of patterning that, according to the founders, makes it possible to bridge across the damage to the parts of the brain that are capable of functioning normally. In documented cases, the children learn to read, write, and do other things that they were thought to never be able to accomplish, and mainly it is a result of the devotion and tireless dedication of their parents.

I am generally attracted to cures like this one and alternative methods in general of approaching illness and disease. Miracles ring true for me. The Institutes for Human Potential saw that treating symptoms was ineffectual (paralysis, mental retardation, seizures, etc.) and led to no progress, whereas treating the source of the problem—an injury somewhere in the brain or central nervous system—was effective and frequently caused a measurable improvement, in which outer symptoms spontaneously disappeared.[1] They pushed for "a true non-surgical approach to the central problem of the brain itself rather than treatment of the periphery wherein the symptoms lay."[2] This approach is of special interest to parents of children with "mental retardation," because as founder Glenn Doman states, "Mental retardation is a symptom and, like most other symptoms, is a symptom of many very different diseases . . . [and] if one successfully attacks the brain injury of which mental retardation can be a symptom, the mental retardation will also disappear spontaneously."[3]

I know from my own work as a healer that anything is possible, and that just because Western medicine doesn't recognize it as "real" doesn't mean a certain "odd" treatment isn't actually more effective than the ones sanctioned by Western doctors and the profit-motivated pharmaceutical industry. In my own healing circles, miracles sometimes happen as a result of drumming, chanting, and hands-on healing without any other treatment. I believe that my method sometimes works for the same reason that the Doman methods work, because I focus on systemic causes rather than peripheral symptoms, giving the immune system a direct boost and stimulating the internal healing mechanisms. In some miraculous way, the symptoms (for instance, a malignant tumor on the pituitary gland) spontaneously disappear.

As a young mother, I found a library copy of Glenn Doman's book *How to Teach Your Baby to Read* and successfully taught reading to my daughter Robyn in the late 1960s.

So when I came across Glenn Doman's name again in this new context of mental retardation after Aaron Eagle was born, I was open to his ideas. His book *What to Do About Your Brain-Injured Child* is a simple handbook of principles and practices for the parent of a child with any one of several injuries (the child may have brain damage, mental retardation, mental deficiency, cerebral palsy, or Down syndrome or be spastic, flaccid, rigid, epileptic, autistic, athetoid, or hyperactive).

At first, Jonathan and I thought maybe we would sometime take Aaron to Philadelphia to the Institutes when he was older, but like so many things in life, the time slipped by without the trip materializing. We learned that there is a significant waiting list, and of course you have to fly there and study. And then you have to spend hours a day actually applying the methods to your child. I should clarify here that when my daughters were born in the late sixties, I was a full-time housewife-mother, and my (first) husband was an officer in the Air Force. At the age of twenty-one, I had a lot of creative energy that channeled happily into stimulating my two young children and dealing responsively with their daily needs. I sewed for my girls, learned gourmet cooking, spent endless hours reading about how to raise them and raising them. I found it interesting work, I felt alive in it, and I didn't have any competing impulses at that point in my life. I learned to structure my time around their naps and bedtime, finding time to read extensively and do the daily chores of attending them.

When Aaron Eagle was born, on the other hand, I was thirty-seven years old and had long been involved in my own very active career in the world. I never intended to stay at home with him past the breast-feeding period, and even then we drove all across the country while I taught workshops and Jonathan kept Aaron, bringing him to me for feedings. And I hate to admit it, but in a certain way, Jonathan and I aren't either one of us very good at following structured regimens of any kind, and now we don't even live in the same house together. I suppose it may be that we are undisciplined, but I also know that we utilize an intuitive or artistic approach to radical learning, with many of the same motivating concepts behind it. I was very impressed with the philosophy behind the policies of the Institutes and the serious dedication required for the parents and kids they take on as their own and to whom they give focused, individualized attention. And I'm in awe of the parents who bring themselves to the task of patterning their children in this method.

I have to say it is a challenge for me to get Aaron Eagle to brush his teeth, take a bath, get dressed, eat meals, and clean up his toys each day. Because I just knew I wasn't going to be the kind of mom who would be able to actually get my child to cross-crawl or "pattern" for sustained periods every day, it was very affirming for me to hear from Dr. Neil Harvey, director of the Institutes, that he understands and finds it acceptable that many people come there and see what they're doing at the Institutes, then go home and integrate whatever they can of the philosophy and practices into their daily lives. They understand that not everyone is suited to the in-house patterning process, yet people can still benefit from their programs and concepts.

From the beginning, we have brought into Aaron's life young, energetic, creative people who are interested and eager to work with him for a reasonable wage as teachers and helpers. The important thing isn't necessarily who spends the whole day stimulating the child with Down syndrome, just that that child gets the necessary stimulation! Of course, as Glenn Doman points out, the parents are going to be especially effective at working with their own child, whom they deeply love. In addition to Jonathan and me, Aaron's older sisters filled that function for a while, as they were in high school and were willing to spend some time each day playing with their little brother. Then when we moved back to the Bay Area from Arizona and Aaron started preschool, we got nannies to come and spend regular hours with him during each week.

Because Jonathan and I were older when Aaron Eagle was born and had already established ourselves in the world as creative artists and healers, we also had the privilege of being able to pay for what we need for Aaron. I never forget this, and I often give thanks for this support in our lives. What would we do, I often wonder, if we were alone in this process, or if we didn't have the money to pay for child care? There are not enough government programs to support parents of disabled children, and the special education

programs vary from city to city, according to the consciousness of the community and the state of its budget. We often
take the line of least resistance and pay for what we need
rather than struggling with bureaucracies and going through
the channels we would have to utilize otherwise.

Aaron Eagle seems to have a special ability to magnetize
the right helpers in his life, people who really like him and
have an abundance of energy and ideas for him. About the
time we started to feel that he needed something individualized, other than preschool, Alejandra Flores came into his
life. Aaron was four years old and had become interested in
basketball. We thought he needed someone to focus on his
particular interests, to challenge him and help him make
progress. I ran a school for healers in Berkeley at the time,
and I was invited to teach in Mexico through a women's
center there, where Alejandra was one of the directors.
Shortly after my visit, she came to the United States to live
for a while and showed up one day at my school. One of
my assistant teachers translated our first conversation.

Alejandra was looking for work and a place to live. I
asked what she did for her work and was amazed to learn
that she had been a special education instructor with four-
year-old children who had Down syndrome! In addition to
these credentials, she had been on the Mexican women's
Olympic basketball team! She moved into an available
room at my school for a time, and in the next few months,
she started learning English and I got a lot of practice
speaking Spanish. Alejandra and Aaron Eagle hit it off

very well, and before long they were playing basketball every day, running regularly, visiting Lake Merritt and the bird sanctuary, doing salsa dancing at La Peña, and other interesting activities.

From the beginning Alejandra focused on Aaron Eagle's sensory-motor development and on stimulating his cardio-vascular system by getting him running, hopping, jumping, climbing, and doing calisthenics, many of the same kinds of activities that would be part of a more formal patterning program. Originally, Aaron had the typical caved-in chest that you can see in many children with Down syndrome, and now he does not. He stooped, and now he does not. He had the "low muscle tone" that describes so many develop-mentally delayed children, and the slow learning that often accompanies it. Alejandra pointed out from the beginning of her time with Aaron Eagle that the daily physical exer-cise she insisted upon fed oxygen to his brain, making him smarter and happier. I learned when I was in Philadelphia that the Doman method, and the work of the Institutes for Human Potential, are more popular and widespread in Mexico and South America than in North America (mainly due to the predictably negative response from the AMA), so it's not surprising that her approach would include con-cepts that no doubt originated with them.

Glenn Doman describes positive physical changes in chil-dren with disabilities who go through the patterning process under the guidance of the Institutes, including growth of the head and chest to normal dimensions; this growth has been true as well for Aaron.[4] And Doman says that, in general, when the Institutes succeeded with brain-injured children, "their bodies became in every way normal." This miracle he attributes to the Institutes' main theorem: that "function determines structure."[5] He said that brain-injured children, as they grew older, tended to grow smaller compared to children their age, because of lack of physical functioning. He used as an example of this natural law any child who becomes seriously ill for a period of time, causing his or her growth to slow down or even temporarily stop. When the child becomes well again, that same child will grow faster until he or she catches up with their peers.[6] So for the brain-injured child, the solution is stimulation, and in order for the stimulus to get to the brain through whatever barrier exists on account of the injury, "You must increase the stimuli in frequency, intensity and duration."[7]

Alejandra has always used this approach with Aaron Eagle, patiently making him repeat physical activities over and over (frequency), assuming that he can learn whatever he practices. If he doesn't pay attention to her request, she says it in a louder voice or forces him to look her straight in the eye (intensity). And she continues the training for weeks and months at a time, until it "takes" (duration). Thanks to his time with Alejandra, Aaron Eagle stands up straight and has become leaner, faster, and taller over the years, his muscles toned. His energy is brighter all the time. He still might prefer to watch a video on television, if he had his way, rather than running around the track. But he never says no to Alejandra and her program of physical training or, for that matter, to her command to wash his own dishes after a meal. When he performs a physical activity, he is much happier for it. Exercise transforms him, as "function determines structure."

Alejandra recently started coaching him for the Special Olympics, since he came of age at his eighth birthday. Whereas he never used to want to run very far, now he can jog around the track three times in a given practice period. She reinforces him with creative amusements, such as the way they stop after a couple of runs around the track and open their arms wide, look at the sky, and exclaim, "What a beautiful sky!" which Aaron Eagle repeats to us with delight. He does abdominal exercises, stretches, and other calisthenics at her direction. And last week he ran his first race in the Alameda County Special Olympics, the smallest boy out there—and the only one in his division! That meant he took home two blue ribbons for first place his first time out.

Frequency, intensity, and duration—these are the all-important principles applied to children learning the intense patterning that stimulates the brain to grow and develop appropriately. The Institutes have amazing and beautiful testimonies of success, although they don't deny their failures. One little girl with Down syndrome, a child of one of their ambassadors to Australia, played the violin at age four and was at the top of her normal classes all through public school. A severely autistic boy went to school and got a Ph.D.

When I was visiting the Institutes, I saw paralyzed children learning to crawl and creep, a young man who had been in a coma moving himself across a mat with enormous effort and personal satisfaction, and babies being held upside down by moms and dads for periods of time. Doman's first priority is getting children onto the floor—out of the cribs, playpens, high chairs, strollers, and other forms of containment that so often restrain and restrict them. On the floor, children (as well as damaged adults) can learn to move instinctually, and when they move, the brain integrates this step in the systematic process of development. If they can't move at all, then they are put on a slant boards so that the movement can happen first by virtue of gravity. The underlying assumption here is that the organism wants to grow and develop, that there is an inbuilt mechanism that will lead even the damaged human toward movement, and eventually walking and talking, and so on. The Institutes have proved this hypothesis over and over again.

I'm sure many parents work with these concepts instinctively, as Jonathan and I did. Aaron Eagle's creeping, crawling, and walking were all events we encouraged for many, many months and celebrated fully when he accomplished them. We let him be on the floor a lot, without diapers as much of the time as possible in our warm Arizona home during the first two years, knowing intuitively that this would lead to his effective mobility. Doman constantly stresses that what helps damaged kids develop normally is to give them unlimited opportunities—the opportunity to creep, crawl, walk, talk, read, and accomplish whatever they might be able to do in life. He thinks parents naturally are capable of presenting these necessary opportunities to their hurt children.

Doman complains about the medical myth that mothers are too emotionally involved to be "objective" about their children and that this makes them "unrealistic." He counters it with his own belief, "There's nobody more realistic than mothers of brain-injured children."[8] He cites the many cases in which it was the parents who pushed for a diagnosis of brain-injury for their child, over and against the judgments of the physician in charge, so that they might get help. And he insists, "Parents are not the problem with children: Parents are the answer."[9] This philosophical stance gives parents permission to have their own authority in relation to what they see and know about their child and to act on their deep beliefs about the child's ability to progress beyond what the doctors have predicted.

In addition to this focused physical time with his tutor, Alejandra, Aaron spends one afternoon after school each week with Alexandra, a former student in the Motherpeace School, who takes him to toy stores for hours at a time, where he studies every single truck, bike, and car in existence. She takes him to cultural events such as dance programs, museums, children's hours, movies, the circus, and to a restaurant where he can indulge his love of homemade french fries. It was Alexandra who took him to play miniature golf one day, and on a whim got him a bucket of balls to shoot at the driving range. What was an experimental gesture on her part has turned into Aaron Eagle's deepest current obsession: golf! Aaron would go golfing every day, if he could only find someone to take him. He turns every stick, pencil, or chopstick into a golf club, and he focuses like a pro. He can take that bucket of balls and spend an hour and a half hitting them across the driving range, just as seriously as the grown-up golfers all around him. He takes his time, practices once or twice for each shot, contemplates the distance, and finally hits that ball down the course.

Perhaps it is our Scottish heritage. When I was a child, I hated golf. All the grown-ups in our family—my grandparents, my father and mother—loved it and played all summer. I thought hitting those little balls across the lawn and then doing all that endless walking to catch up to them was the ultimate in labor-intensive boredom. I never developed any skill at it, nor any attraction to it. Now I watch this boy of mine take to it like a duck to water, and I have to smile in appreciation. He loves it so much, I'll probably have to learn it, after a lifetime of avoidance! Lately it's been raining a lot, and Aaron Eagle is heartbroken—no golfing. Yesterday Alexandra had to take him to Toys-R-Us to shoot baskets for two hours instead.

Another babysitter, Debbie, takes Aaron on the bus to places like Lake Anza in Tilden Park (an urban recreation area in the East Bay) and Fairy Land (a children's playland) in Oakland. They visit the University of California campus and join in with the conga drummers who meet on the plaza every weekend. Or they get honey-sweetened frozen yogurt and then walk across town at a leisurely pace, taking buses for the fun of it and ending up somewhere later in the day for brown rice and tofu, another of Aaron's favorites! If this sounds unstructured, you simply have to think of all the life skills that are dealt with in the course of these ordinary activities: crossing the street, paying with money for a frozen yogurt, learning to interact socially, learning to orient geographically, walking long distances, taking buses, and so on.

In special education, this focus on ordinary activities is called "life skills," and they are taught with the hope that the child will eventually become at least partially independent in his or her life. We try to provide a variety of life activities for Aaron Eagle, those that he reaches for himself from his own motivation, and those that we think are necessary stimuli for his development and growth toward independence in his life. As the years go by, Aaron Eagle seems happier and healthier in every way, and I cannot imagine this is not related to these natural, creative, and very human opportunities we provide for him. Every month, he moves toward more experiences of real independence.

He is getting old enough that we can begin to take him places where stimulation is the thing. I recently took him to visit the Exploratorium in San Francisco, where there are so many buttons to push in order to make interesting things happen that Aaron couldn't believe he was allowed to touch them. He ran nervously from one thing to the next, until he began to understand that it was okay for him to press buttons, turn levers, pull handles, put his hands in bubbly liquids, and all other manner of sensory stimulation. We sat across from each other wearing a double set of microphones and earphones that allowed us to hear our voices amplified, and then pushed buttons to make the pitch higher or lower and the speed faster or slower. He loved it!

We have the Lawrence Hall of Science here in Berkeley, a place where kids can go to learn about things and make things happen. And there are children's Saturday morning programs with musicians and puppeteers that Aaron enjoys very much. All this contributes a great deal to his sense of freedom and exploration, to his sensate pleasure, and to his ability to interact with other children as well. Perhaps families who have a child with Down syndrome and other siblings arrive at these high levels of stimulation and interaction more casually and without so much intention, but with an only child, we have to think about it to make it happen.

Aaron Eagle likes having control over his life. He likes making choices. He has certain associations with each person in his life that he asks for routinely. "I want Debbie, bus, beach," he will say one day; and "I want Alexandra, golfing, toy store," on another day. If possible, we let him have his way, or we teach him to understand how many days it will be before that particular thing can happen. He is an urban boy at core, with friends all over the city who recognize him and ask after him. He has restaurants where the waiters and waitresses know him, places where he can talk them into giving him a frozen yogurt for free, and a french-fry chef at the Rockridge Cafe who has given Aaron two of his own hats already.

The only problem we seem to have with Aaron's activities is his own resistance to learning something new. He often balks at the idea of doing something different or something he hasn't done before. I've taken to getting down eye-to-eye with him and saying, "Aaron, you don't understand this, because you've never seen it before, so you need to trust us on it. We think you will like it if you try it." On a good day, he will agree.

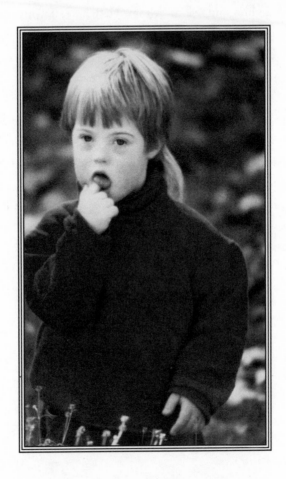

Aaron Eagle in nature, age seven.
Photo by Jonathan Tenney.

Chapter Seven

Trusting Psychic
Perception

꙳

W HEN I WAS GROWING UP, THE SO-CALLED psychic, or invisible, levels of contact and connection were rarely mentioned or acknowledged in our family or among my friends. As children we were interested in psychic games; for instance, I remember experiments in which I was able, without looking, to feel a friend's finger coming close to the skin on my back before it reached me physically. And I was indelibly impressed one night in high school when my sister was involved in a bad car accident and ended up in a coma for several hours and my father sat bolt upright in bed at the moment that the accident happened and before the police called our house. But we never discussed it or asked questions about how it worked.

I began my psychic studies, long before Aaron Eagle came into my life, in 1976 during my own shamanic healing crisis. A shamanic healer is a person who is magically healed of illness or disease and then "called" to be a healer for others. There is almost always a crisis of health or near-death, which is accompanied by visions and involuntary psychic experiences and leads to a manifested healing talent that becomes available in the person healed. Like classic shamans in other cultures more tribal than ours, I healed myself of physical illness without intervention by Western medicine. During the same period of time, I co-created the Motherpeace Tarot Cards with Karen Vogel and wrote *Motherpeace: A Way to the Goddess Through Magic, Art, and Tarot*. The tradition of Tarot depends on faculties that Western culture define as paranormal, providing information not generally available to the ordinary, rational consciousness. Therefore a Tarot reader is said to be able to "divine" the future, or see into the hidden realities.

The psychic faculties that I developed over a period of fifteen years have come in very handy in my relationship with Aaron Eagle. Much of the time my approach with him simply defies rational definition (as he himself so often does). There are so many times when the direct, "normal" approach fails to elicit the desired response from him. Other times I am away from home, absent from him physically, yet our contact is viable and strong through other than ordinary channels. He may not always want to talk on the telephone, but he is remarkably available across the psychic pathways.

I can't really say whether his extreme sensitivity on this level is related to Down syndrome, and if others with his condition share his special talent for responding to the invisible world. Aaron has always talked to spirits (or at any rate, to something we can't see that we imagine as spirits), and he seems to react and respond to communications that take place in what Australian aboriginal people have named the Dreamtime. When Aaron was barely able to stand up, he used to spend time in front of the mirror shaking a gourd rattle as though he knew what he was doing, looking exactly like a tribal medicine man at work expelling the demons. He would turn to us and "heal" us with the rattle. Even though I know he was "playing" and probably imitating something he had seen someone else doing, still in the back of my mind, I couldn't help but wonder if he was bringing something through from another lifetime or tapping into some other level of experience or knowledge.

Aaron has deep feelings and reactions to things that are going on around him, which sometimes upset him in ways he cannot describe or tell us about. At those times, his behavior doesn't seem to match whatever the current situation is, as if there is something happening at a deeper level than the rational. For example, he might feel insecure, or have sad or negative experiences that seem unrelated to present time. He might be listless or lose his appetite, act sleepy and lethargic for no apparent reason, cry a lot over small things, and basically communicate an emotional distress through his body rather than being able to tell us what's upsetting him.

Fortunately, I am very intuitive, so a lot of my communication with Aaron is naturally on that invisible level. I tend to get flashes when he's feeling sad or confused about something that happened at school or something with me and his daddy. If Aaron is having some experience that strikes me as incongruous, I will sometimes get right down at his level and look him in the eye and try to name the problem by amplifying what I see as the symptomatic expression of it. In Arnold Mindell's model, called "process psychology," this activity of mine is defined as bringing the "secondary" (invisible) process up into the "primary" (visible) conversation.[1] I get a hunch about what is "really" going on, and I try it out on Aaron by naming it, or naming his behavior. I might say something like, "You look really sad," or "It seems like something happened that made you mad," or something of that sort. Especially when he was very young, I would work hard to get eye contact to happen so that he could read the messages behind my words, because the words alone seemed too complicated for him.

I remember the excitement I felt the first time I stumbled across this method and successfully made a communication with him. He was reacting in a way that didn't really make sense to me, getting really mad about some toy that wouldn't do what he wanted. I had never seen him act that way before about a physical object, and it seemed like some kind of transference. I suddenly had a hunch that his immediate upset was related to something else entirely, so I shifted things with him very directly. I began to talk about the fight that his dad and I had had in very clear, direct, simple language, saying that I thought he must be feeling sad because of it. In order to do this, I had to validate my own paranormal or "psychic" information in that moment and then act from there. Once I had his undivided attention, because I had named the real problem and it resonated within him, I could ask him about it, and he could cry and release his feelings.

I have kept that approach in mind since then, and it always works. He seems very grateful to be truly seen and understood, and I feel our telepathic closeness and it makes me happy. Together we break through the apparent barrier created by his handicap. After one of these occasions, he truly feels better and acts different, so I know it is not my imagination at work. He also seems to like having emotions, and having them named. Once we introduced the concept of being mad or sad, he made pictures of both states, and he announces now when he's mad or happy or sad.

As a mother, one always has to check out the imagination and compare it to reality. So many fears and doubts come up and can get in the way of our natural intuitive abilities. When Aaron was in first grade and having quite a bad year at school for a variety of reasons, there was one teacher aide in the special education room whose behavior I didn't like in relation to the kids. One day I requested that this particular aide not be allowed to work with Aaron, telling the director very clearly what I felt about the person's "negative energy." Unfortunately, it's quite common for people to think a person who talks about somebody's "energy" is paranoid or having a fantasy, and the director must have felt this way about me that day. She failed to take me seriously, and nothing was actually done to get a different person to be with Aaron Eagle.

The very next day there was a dramatic incident at school that proved me correct in my perceptions and necessitated the immediate discharge of the teacher aide from Aaron's school site. I never got all the precise details, but the gist of it was that the person lost her temper and yelled at Aaron Eagle quite uncontrollably, right in front of everyone on the playground during recess. Aaron, quite innocent of any misbehavior, was devastated by the attack, and the school had to notify me of the incident. It was embarrassing to the director, and other teachers who had overheard my appraisal of the situation the day before, because I had clearly seen something that was about to manifest as trouble, and they had chosen to ignore it. I suppose it was somewhat ironic for them that the incident should have involved my child, rather than someone else's, so that I had to be informed about it.

I learned to trust my own perceptions about Aaron Eagle through trial and error. There was a period of time when he was approaching his fifth birthday during which he and I were not getting along. It's the only time this has ever happened, and it was terribly disconcerting for me. I couldn't really believe it, but for a few months, it seemed as if Aaron didn't like me much, and it hurt my feelings very deeply. I kept trying to work on myself—refining my reactions, telling myself he's only a little hurt boy, that he couldn't help how he was acting, and so on. Although that was true, my feelings were still hurt, and the situation was becoming emotionally charged for me. I felt rejected by my own son.

I tried every form of verbal communication. I tried humor, being detached, and not taking his behavior seriously. I attempted to make light of the way he wouldn't relate to me and didn't seem to care about me. I tried to ignore it and just keep acting normal. There was a coldness and disconnectedness in his behavior toward me that, in a normal person, I would attribute to their being very deeply angry at me. After a few weeks of this, it became a crisis for me. I went to Aaron one night when I was putting him to bed and cried, the way I would share my feelings with someone my age or my equal. I told him he was hurting my feelings, that my heart hurt, and that I needed him to be more loving with me. Still no response.

I was desperate. I gave up trying to get Aaron to respond and began to pray about it, asking the Mother for help. I got the idea of creating a wonderful birthday for Aaron. I set my will to it, applying creative focus to the event, preparing a party that he could have at preschool with his little friends. I took birthday hats, cake, frozen yogurt, and party favors to school, along with a babysitter of Aaron's whom I hired to go as a clown. It was a wonderful event, and all the children were pleased to be part of it.

Aaron got to be the center of attention, and at one point he broke all our hearts by going slowly and poignantly around the table and giving a personalized greeting to each individual child. He understood for the first time that the party was for him; it was his birthday.

Then I went home and spent the day in a state of total focus on Aaron and my own prayers for his fifth birthday. I gathered a stack of magazines and cut out pictures that reminded me of him and of all the things I hoped and dreamed would come to him in the next year. I found pictures of children playing on playground equipment, a boy sitting at a desk reading a book, a potty, a playhouse, a boy running, another one playing a banjo, a clown, and many other interesting and optimistic images. I found old postcards with pictures of power animals to help him, Goddesses to watch over and protect him, and pictures of mommies and daddies with happy little children. Then when he came home that evening, I showed him the pictures, and I started to place them on a large sheet of poster board, like a collage.

After Aaron went to bed that night, I spent four uninterrupted hours putting the collage together, bringing my prayers to life. The activity itself was enjoyable, sacred, and transformative. I knew I was engaged in an act of magic, and I didn't stop until it was finished. When Aaron woke up the next day, our conflict was over. I am not exaggerating. The terrible tension between us was released. Not a trace of it remained, and it has never returned in that intense, unresolvable way. I will probably never know what caused our estrangement in the first place, and I can't say that I rationally understand the mechanisms for healing it. It was a badly needed miracle, and I was very grateful for what I can only assume was help from the spirits. My prayers were heard and answered, and my relationship with my special son was restored in beauty.

Aaron was delighted when he saw what I had made for him. We named every picture on the board, and he laughed and chattered about it, showing it to everyone who came around to visit. The completed collage was pleasing visually to both of us, and I had it mounted and shrink-wrapped like a work of art, so that it would be more or less permanent. It hangs on the wall in Aaron's bedroom, and it is a special object between us that, whenever we talk about it together, rekindles that moment of reunion. It stands as a witness to the depth of our relationship and reminds me that we can handle anything if my heart stays open to him.

I remember that, as my daughters grew up, there came a time when I had to teach them to honor their intuitive abilities. I knew as they moved away from my protective wing and began to make their own choices and actions in the world, they needed to know the spiritual secret to successful living: one must be able to hear one's own inner voice. It was a concept that I taught to them, assuring them that they would be glad at learning to follow their own guidance from within. But Aaron doesn't seem to really understand very many concepts, so the situation with him is quite different. I find that he is so naturally open to an intuitive way of being in the world that I have to learn to simply be intuitive, rather than analyze it or think about it or even practice it. Aaron has sensitized me to a further refinement of the intuition: that not only can a person hear his or her own inner voice, but he can also hear mine, and I can hear his!

I considered this understanding of mine to be a private one, personal and unique to my relationship with my special son, until I was given an unpublished paper presented at a conference, "Treatments and Research of Experienced Anomalous Trauma," in Santa Fe, in March 1993. The presentation was by a doctor, Rima Laibow, about one of her clients, Eve, a girl who had been diagnosed as severely autistic and mute, and whose silence was miraculously broken at age fourteen by her mother. The mother, Brigette Hanf, told how in a "rage of despair" she handed her daughter a pen and paper and demanded that she write her name. Eve wrote her name, which was her first verbal communication in fourteen years of "total passivity."

What's fascinating in Eve's story (which the mother told at the conference) is that as communication between mother and child opened up, it revealed that Eve had secretly taught herself to read at the age of four and could read any book in their library, including great literature (Shakespeare, Dostoevsky, T. S. Eliot) and books in foreign languages. Eve's memories, which she wrote down verbatim, included ". . . her birth, names and street addresses of people we had known in England where we had been living, literal transcripts of conversations overheard years ago, poems, essays on the books we had read to her, much of it interspersed with words, phrases and sentences in French, Italian and German, even bits of Latin and Yiddish, none of which were spoken at home. All were correctly spelled."[2]

Because of her apparent "autism," Eve's brilliance had been overlooked and was naturally doubted by authorities of all kinds—doctors, therapists, teachers, schools—who simply denied that her reported talents were possible, given her affliction. The school believed Eve's mother to be the "author" of the writings. (The mother mentions that even now her relatives are still not speaking to her because they believe her to be mad for having such wild ideas about her daughter's possibilities.) Yet she forged ahead, alone believing in her "handicapped" daughter, just the way so many mothers have had to do. The extremely shy Eve finally agreed to demonstrate her private abilities for school authorities. In front of the strongly doubting school principal, the testing psychologist, and the supervisor of special education, Eve—by herself, alone at a work table— "racked up a perfect score. Staff filed out in silence. Their single comment, weeks later, was, 'We saw it but we can't explain it.'"[3] Happily, Eve ended up at Camp Hill school in Pennsylvania, where she is understood and appreciated by the staff and can learn in her own very special ways.

The Eve story is pertinent to my story because the mother, Brigitte Hanf, speaks at length, quoting her daughter's writings, about the psychic connection between them and the actual pain and confusion it caused the daughter to be able to feel and know the mother's thoughts. I have always felt that Aaron Eagle was visibly affected by the worries, doubts, fears, hidden angers, feelings, and so forth, of me and his daddy, as well as his caretakers and others. Many people, when I mention this, feel that I'm making it up or imagining it, believing that such interconnectedness is impossible or at least overstated. Yet I see it over and over again, and feel certain it is true. Brigitte Hanf's paper corroborates my experience by quoting from the "horse's mouth," that is, her daughter Eve's own explanation.

Ms. Hanf tells about a walk she took with her daughter one day, after which they went in the house and Eve sat down and wrote, "You are wondering if I am noticing the daffodils." Her very surprised mother agreed, and then Eve continued, "I get thoughts from feeling great tension coming from you . . . but western famished world won't address road to words by ESP." The shocked mother begins to have "thought conversations" with her damaged daughter, only to have revealed the hidden dimensions of their deep mother-child bond.

> Gradually, as Eve's reports on my inner life became more explicit, I began to fear for my own balance. More than once in the night I found her sobbing from my nightmares. On mornings after I'd been out for dinner, she would repeat the contents of the previous evening's dinner conversation. When I was ill

in hospital, she at home got frantic at "seeing" the
medical procedures I was undergoing.[4]

I too have heard Aaron Eagle making difficult sounds in
the night indicating stress or tension after I have had a particularly harsh nightmare or a waking fight with someone.
She concludes, probably feeling too much guilt, the way
mothers are prone to do, "So here was an answer to the
moody, seizure prone, bed wetting, obsessive behaviour
these many years. It had to do, evidently, with mother—
and others—having thoughts and dreams which were upsetting further an already precarious equilibrium."[5]

Of course, all psychic gifts have a good side to them as
well as the horrific oversensitivities, and Eve's is no excep-
tion. Her mother describes her ability to hold an object (a
belt buckle given to her mother as a gift) and tell everything about it, including its Indian maker and the tribe he
came from, who bought it, the story behind it, and so on.
(In Western psychic schools, this ability is called "psy-
chometry" and is often used by police departments and private investigators, who hire psychics to help find lost or
stolen articles or people.) Eve writes about her anger and
frustration being born cesarean, having a fetal monitor
used on her, being separated from her mother at birth, and
other minute details. Glenn Doman, from the Institutes for
Human Potential, states that their share of children born
by cesarean section is about three times normal, which
could either produce the brain injury or be the result of it.[6]

Hanf writes:

> All children, as is now understood, are born with a
> highly developed sensitivity to the tangible and in-
> tangible life without and within themselves. The
> child with autism, and some others, for some reason
> genetic or otherwise, has retained his original vul-
> nerability. Because he is so fearfully unable to layer
> himself with the protective clothing of acceptable so-
> cial mores his only alternative must be self isolation.
> As for the rest of us, perhaps it is time to recognize
> how far we have gone to the other extreme in our
> denial of what we choose to call the paranormal.[7]

I hate to think about how many children are in pain because we—their parents—are unaware of how our thoughts
and feelings affect them in their enormous, unacknowledged sensitivity. As we understand more about these unde-
niable psychic links in understanding and communication,
we can use them to our advantage for helping to further
strengthen the contact between us and our children. I have
come to rely on these invisible threads of connection between me and Aaron Eagle. I see them working in our lives,
whether we like it or not, whether anyone else believes in
them or not.

Aaron Eagle has always been responsive to the hidden or
unspoken tensions among people, and he frequently attempts
to break the tension and bring things back to harmony. In
large groups, he will often create a bond that unites all the

people by going around a dinner table and giving each person a hug. His tenderness opens hearts and changes the energy in the room. His freedom to spontaneously reach out and love everyone equally is undeniably healing to all of us. His sensitivity is unmatched.

Last fall I decided to travel away from the country for a whole month. This is longer than I had ever previously been away from Aaron Eagle, and although he was going to be happily spending the time with his daddy, still I worried and prayed over the length of my absence, asking for help from the invisible realm. I knew it was crucial that I feel good about the journey, and I trusted that both of us could manage it without damage. Just as Eve's mother realized, any unnecessary worry and guilt is harmful, rather than helpful, to the situation. I believed Aaron was old enough to handle my time away, and I determined to act on that belief.

I made several telephone calls from Greece to Aaron's house during the first two weeks of my trip, and each time Aaron was fine, happily describing his day at school or playing with his trucks or whatever was current. On the morning of the third week away (exactly the amount of time I had ever stayed away from him in the past), I awoke from a disturbing nightmare in which Aaron was my puppy and he and I had decided in some sort of ritualistic way that he was to take a potion and die. In the dream there was no emotion as I held the puppy on my lap, he simply took the poison and began to throw up as planned, and I knew he was dying. Suddenly I felt my intense love for him, and I held him tight and said over and over, "Aaron Eagle, I love you so much, I love you so much."

When I woke up, I tried to figure out why I would dream that Aaron was a puppy, and why he would die in the dream, and what could be wrong. Upset and worried, I called home to daddy's house, but I only got a machine. Next I called Karen Vogel at my house, because she was to be having Aaron stay overnight once each week during the duration of my travels. I described the dream and asked Karen what she thought it could mean. She said, "I wasn't going to tell you until you got home, but Jonathan cut off Aaron's tail."

Suddenly, I knew what the dream was about. Haircutting, in dreams, represents and/or precedes initiation in many cultures. I had been growing Aaron's hair in a "tail" (my puppy) since he was a baby, and it was halfway down his back. Sometimes I would braid it for special occasions. Once or twice, Jonathan and I had discussed cutting the tail, because he thought it was a bit feminine. I always clung to it, feeling that Aaron didn't mind, and that it was very beautiful on him. So while I was gone for a month, his daddy had taken the liberty of cutting off the tail without having to work it out with me. The event seemed to signify the end of Aaron's babyhood (the death of my puppy) and my maternal attachment to him, and seen in that light the dream held deep meaning. Although I was pretty mad at his dad for making such a unilateral decision in my absence, I also saw the whole event as magical and sacred beyond our egos.

After that, I called Aaron's tutor, Alejandra Flores, to get her feedback about the dream, and she told me that Aaron had indeed been sick and throwing up for two days, but she thought he was basically okay and going back to school that day. The fact that in the dream Aaron Eagle and I had agreed, ritually, to this death of his identity made me feel that we had made a joint psychic decision that he could be a "big boy" and get along without me for a whole month, longer than either of us had ever been challenged to do without each other before. When I arrived home and saw little Aaron without his tail, I felt crushed and disappointed over the loss, but I also saw that he was more integrated and well than he had ever been before when I had returned from being away. We had truly been through the fires of Initiation together, and all but the haircutting and the illness had taken place on the unseen level.

In all relationships, this psychic or paranormal level of communication serves a healing and connecting function. But between me and Aaron Eagle I especially treasure it, because it so often makes up for the lack of the ordinary communication that would take place with a "normal" child. These psychic talks he and I have satisfy a need in me to feel connected at deep levels with those I love. It is not Aaron's way to state in words his deep feelings of love and caring but rather to show them through body language or, even more simply, to demonstrate them through his good health and well-being.

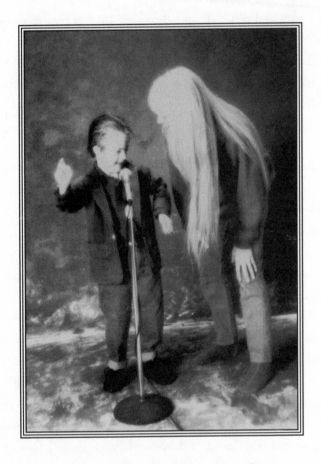

Aaron Eagle at microphone with Vicki.
Photo by Irene Young.

Chapter Eight

Mainstreaming
Independence

ॐ

I'VE ALWAYS WONDERED IF AARON EAGLE KNOWS he's different, and if so, what he thinks about it. I thought I saw him comprehend it once when he was trying to learn to crawl. I either perceived or imagined his existential angst as he struggled to make his body do what his mind knew was possible. I've heard it said that one of the difficult things for people with Down syndrome is that they gradually are able to understand the situation—that they are different, slower, disabled in some way—and have to integrate this knowledge. A psychic once told us that Aaron's destiny in the world was connected to this painful, conscious knowledge of his own condition. Because he would be aware of his own condition, she said, he would be able to help others who have Down syndrome with issues of self-esteem and personal worth.

Jason Kingsley, a young man with Down syndrome who has appeared on "Sesame Street" and other television shows, and whose mother, Emily Kingsley, wrote a made-for-TV movie called *Kids Like These,* sums up the problem: "I just can't handle it, I just can't handle hard things," he exclaims, adding that he still "has a lot of pain. . . . It takes such a long time . . . to learn."[1] "I'm sick of all this Down syndrome stuff," he adds. The higher the ability to function, the more likely the person with Down syndrome is to contact feelings of frustration, disappointment, the body's lack of ability to keep up with the brain, and so on. Like all other people with disabilities, a person with Down syndrome has to learn to work with what's available and do without the rest. It takes constant courage for a disabled person to go the extra mile, to try hard to do the same thing everybody else does without thinking. That's why society needs to supply so much more support and cooperation for people with handicaps. Recent legislation forcing businesses to make themselves wheelchair accessible, for example, is necessary in a society that won't otherwise take the needed extra steps to accommodate people with disabilities.

People with disabilities are pushing for their ultimate independence. The Center for Independent Living here in Berkeley has pioneered the concept, creating a workable model for the rest of the country. The model is based on mobility and inclusion in society. It is commonplace here to see people with various states of paralysis going down the street in their electric wheelchairs, making their way about town, talking through specially developed tubes hooked up to their chairs, enabling them to go shopping, get the mail, go to work, drive cars, and do many of the things that the rest of us rely on as part of our definition of "normal." The movies *My Left Foot* and *Gabby* illustrated this agenda with their main characters with cerebral palsy who were able to paint and type with the toes of their feet and thereby enter the world of normal human communication and interaction.

In a certain sense, and not without justification, the effort to achieve some modicum of equality for people with disabilities has necessitated an emphasis on normalizing them. They pretty much have to learn to behave as the rest of us do, in order to be included in our scene. Fortunately, there has recently been an effort to normalize the environment for their use as well, which seems a good transition. Requiring that all commercial businesses in a town be wheelchair accessible, for example, is an enormous transformation of society in the interest of bringing people with disabilities into the common areas, rather than attempting to get them to somehow become enough like the rest of us that they can get around.

I had some discomfort with this agenda for Aaron Eagle, because I was afraid it meant molding him into a docile American citizen who could at best one day work somewhere like McDonald's. It didn't strike me as being in his (or my) interest for him to strive to be "normal," since most so-called normal people holding down normal jobs don't seem happy or fulfilled. Even for my "retarded" son, I had higher aspirations than for him to be doling out processed, frozen, chemical-laden "fast food" at slave wages in a fast-food joint.

Then one day I switched on his television set, and while I waited for the channels to change from TV to VCR, a McDonald's commercial came on. A young man with Down syndrome was turning burgers, smiling brightly. I was so moved just to see a differently-abled person in prime-time television advertising, I cried. It was uncanny that my verbatim thoughts should have been turned into reality like that before my eyes. Media complicates things terrifically, in terms of our being able to figure out what's really happening. The boy on the television screen who had Down syndrome was genuinely happy flipping burgers, but then he was actually working at being an actor, which might be a pretty interesting job (a glamour job) for anybody. Yet I was emotionally touched by the scene of a "retarded" person working in the normal world. I felt grateful that he was participating visibly.

All children need to be supported and nurtured in the direction that their inborn talents naturally take them. But for how many children in America is this the norm? If genetically abnormal children with a "handicap" can thrive and achieve miraculous success in mainstream society, the way Chris Burke of TV's "Life Goes On" has, for example, what might be possible for all the so-called normal children if they were actually nourished like the young and vital beings that they are? Americans put such a premium on having children turn out "normal" that it's easy to stunt their growth at every unusual turn in their lives. As if growing a Japanese bonsai tree, we feel compelled to prune them and keep them small, growing within the boundaries we have imagined for them. Our children are capable of so much more than we allow them to achieve, and for children with handicaps the assumptions about them are serious obstacles to their actual individuation.

Nigel Hunt, an English boy with Down syndrome, wrote himself a wonderfully inspiring and entertaining story in 1967. His father wrote a preface in which he gave his own version of Nigel's story. Nigel's father, Douglas Hunt, describes Nigel as a "mongol," using the standard lexicon of the time and says that Nigel wrote the book himself in "his own unaided and spontaneous effort" after his father showed him only how to use the shift key for capital letters on the typewriter. Douglas Hunt discusses the experts and their "preconceived ideas of what 'these children' can do. They do not easily admit that they have underestimated them."[2]

Nigel's father describes Nigel's many ideal school situations; he was treated as a fully integrated participant in the classes with normal children, and he was given every opportunity to learn whatever he was capable of. He calls the book "an epoch-making book because it may encourage other parents or teachers who have children like Nigel to deal with."[3] Nigel's mother had originally taught him to read using pictures of each word, somewhat like the flash card method recommended by Glenn Doman in *How to Teach Your Baby to Read*. His father tells the story of Nigel hearing the word *mongol* and going next door to his grandmother to ask what it meant. She responded that a Mongol was an inhabitant of Mongolia.[4]

Professor Hunt mentions that for two years, to their "subsequent deep regret," they sent Nigel to a special school for "educationally subnormal children," where he associated with children "considerably more retarded than he and was constantly told, 'No, you can't do that, Nigel; that's too difficult for you.'" When they saw how negatively this was affecting Nigel, they placed him in a private school where he received "strict and loving discipline and excellent teaching." "'Problem,' is the word; not 'tragedy,'" he goes on, adding that Nigel brought them "untold joy."[5] I was very amused to read in his father's piece that Nigel can go into any shop in London and come out with whatever he went there for, but—like Aaron Eagle—"often with a little extra gift as well."[6]

Before the completion of Nigel's book, his mother died, which was a great loss to both father and son. Douglas Hunt tells of Nigel's gradual acceptance of his mother's death, because he could see her and knew that "she [was] still with him, but in a different way." Father and son went to live at one of the Camp Hill Villages, where "there is not distinction between the mentally handicapped and the 'normal' workers and their families, who live in the villages just as do the others," where they lived a "happy but busy communal life."[7] In showing the book to Nigel, along with the foreword written by another professor, the father learned the answer to a question he had posed, the same question I have asked about Aaron Eagle: Does Nigel know about himself, does he have self-awareness of his handicap? And the answer was yes, that he had "long ago accepted the fact of his mental handicap." And their time at Camp Hill Village allowed this to become more healthily integrated; as the "resident villagers" there who shared a house with the Hunts would say: "This is our village, because we are handicapped."[8]

Surely every soul has a destiny, and each child has talents and skills that can develop into something special and unique that will make that human being's life a worthwhile and meaningful one. When a child loves music, that child needs to sing; when she's visual, she needs to paint; when he's agile, he needs to learn to turn somersaults. The Huichol Indians in Mexico assume that most people in their culture will either be artists or shamans. When a child begins to show a tendency in one direction or another, that child is given opportunities to learn a craft and follow a path "to completion." The tribal life revolves around art and ceremony, and the sacred is never perceived as separate from what one does with one's life.

As soon as the need for money was introduced into Huichol culture, this idyllic structure began to crack and give way to economic priorities. What about America? Our main goal is to make enough money, even though these days almost nobody can do it. Things cost so much, it's impossible for the average family to get by on what even two parents make, and most families don't even have two parents anymore. Families who have a child with Down syndrome feel the extra stresses and demands of raising that special child, frequently at the same time as other children with their own needs. What talents are lying dormant in the many special children growing up in America right now? How many young artists, musicians, actors, ministers, writers, and craftspeople are missing their chance to express themselves right this minute, as they are herded through poorly funded special education programs in the public school system?

The parents of special children have consistently shown that they know how to beat the system, how to make a difference, and how to empower themselves and their children in the process. I am now one of this active group of citizens, and I have to thank Aaron Eagle for forcing me to be a parent who participates in the educational process! He awakened in me the need to take action and engage with society in a responsible way. I see that if we don't look out for our kids, truly no one else will. I think of Barbara Lubin, a local activist and mother of Charlie Lubin, her son with Down syndrome. When my daughters (now twenty-four and twenty-six) were growing up in Berkeley in the 1970s, they were in a theater group with Charlie Lubin, so I was particularly touched to learn Barbara's story.

In an interview with Penny Rosenwasser, Barbara described how Charlie went every day for twelve years around the corner to the neighborhood drugstore, where there was a soda fountain, to sit on the same stool each day and order the same lunch: tuna, chips, and a Coke.[9] Meanwhile, Barbara had what the parents of children with disabilities have come to know as "respite time"—that desperately needed break from the high-intensity focus of relating to the needs of a special child. One day Charlie came home and said they were selling Ozzie's, the soda fountain. Barbara learned that speculators had bought the store to turn a profit, and she subsequently went to bat for Charlie, the community, the owner of the soda fountain, and by extension every local merchant in Berkeley.

She successfully raised money, obtained signatures, and won the first commercial rent control agreement in the country (which was later rescinded by the courts). And she went on from that experience in local politics to get on the school board, and finally to getting the concept of mainstreaming into the public school system in such a way that the whole country could use the model. Barbara Lubin empowered herself, her children, and her community in response to the needs of her very special child, Charlie, and her story is not so different from hundreds of other stories from parents of children with disabilities or mental retardation. It's Artemis, the Mama Bear, fighting with her life and overcoming all opponents for the sake of her cubs and what they need. Now Charlie is grown up, and he holds down an independent job bagging groceries at a local Safeway store.

Every day, he does something that requires skill and earns him a good wage, and he gets to be genuinely social, the way many people with Down syndrome like to be.

What used to be called mainstreaming by the special education people when they wanted to discuss the most progressive, up-to-date ways of approaching disabled students is now known as "inclusion." Generally speaking, the best option for Aaron is to be around "normal" or nondisabled children as much as possible, since he tends to imitate the behavior of others. He learns the songs, words, sports, games, and movements of regular kids. Like a mime, Aaron Eagle looks at something or someone, takes it all in, and then brings it back out through his own body. But when he spends his time with normal children, it's also difficult for him to make a close friend, because they stay separate from him, feeling him to be a bit strange; he also learns not-so-useful things, such as pointing objects at other people as if they are guns, sticking out his tongue at his teacher, sexism, racism, and so forth. When he is fully integrated into normal children's activities, I fear that he will miss out on being with other children like himself. And when he is in special education classes, I fear he will become more disabled by association. It's an unending dilemma.

Special education is only a microcosm of the larger culture and its many dysfunctional institutions. As in all American institutions, certain values hold sway, and others are given short shrift. For me—an alternative healer, a radical feminist, and always a rebellious and iconoclastic parent—

the system has many obvious flaws. But it's the only game in town. What it always boils down to is miracles and special people. It is necessary to deconstruct the impersonalness of the system and replace it with whatever personal contact is possible. The success of every program depends on so many variables, it's hard to have much control over any of it. Yet whenever Jonathan or I consider any other living situations, or work opportunities that would take us to another place, one of the items we have to consider is where Aaron Eagle would go to school and whether there is a decent program for him.

Aaron's first integrated experience was a preschool program in Oakland where he was racially and culturally mixed with all kinds of other kids. His attendance at the school was paid for by state funds channeled through Alameda County, and his experience was exceptionally good. The special education person was a specialist, with a child of her own with Down syndrome as well, and she used active sign language and helped Aaron make headway in his communications. When Aaron turned three, however, the laws required that he had to move into the public school system, where he became the responsibility of the City of Oakland.

Jonathan and I went through what all parents of children with disabilities have come to know as the IEP, the Individualized Educational Plan, for our particular child. Parents meet with "specialists" like speech therapists, psychologists, special education teachers, and workers from the school district to determine what particular things Aaron Eagle needs in order to develop his potential and how we can best meet those needs. The IEP is crucial to the child's successful entry into the public school system; whatever it says the child needs, the school system is mandated to provide. It is for parents a means of putting leverage on an otherwise not very interested system in order to accomplish the stated goals. After the IEP is signed and delivered, the school district has an obligation by law to perform whatever tasks are necessary to fulfill the directions written there.

I was quite impressed when first introduced to this procedure and couldn't help wondering what school would have been like for my normal children if there had been such a plan of action for them! I think all children should be dealt with as if they have needs that can be legally mandated. The only real mandate I know about for normal kids is that they are required to attend school, no matter how boring or irrelevant it is. I used to convince my girls they should stay in school, not because school had much going for it creatively, but because I knew they would find it more difficult to cope on the outside than they would by going the normal (but often quite dull) route of getting a diploma.

But the problem with the IEP process is that it is twisted into local politics and all kinds of issues that don't really have much to do with individual children. So placements are made that don't necessarily comply with the requirements of the IEP, and things have to be fought constantly; time and energy have to be expended in order to stay with the process and make sure that the child's needs are in fact met. Fighting the school district on behalf of your special child is enormously time-consuming and draining, although it does ultimately seem to pay off. I've seen some warrior-parents at work over the years who successfully fought uphill battles for their kids that required them to go through lawyers and courtroom scenes until things changed for the better.

When Aaron Eagle received his first public school placement, we were warned behind the scenes that the school chosen for him wasn't right for him. His IEP said he must have "full inclusion" or the "least restrictive environment" possible, and instead he was assigned to a restricted special education classroom (no normal kids). We took him to school there one day and left him, against our better judgment. The kids were watching television when we dropped Aaron off, and when we picked him up at the end of the morning, we didn't even discuss bringing him back. There was a kind of gray aura in the whole place, depressing and uninteresting.

Rather than go through the inevitable fight, which we had also been advised about, we just called around town to see if there were any private preschools that would take a child with Down syndrome. Most said no, that they lacked the "proper" training, but finally Big Trees Montessori School in Berkeley said yes, and we enrolled him for a probationary period of two weeks. It was such a relief to hear somebody relate to our problem without a big charge of unnecessary concern. The openhearted director simply responded to my question by saying, "Well, I don't see why not," and that was that. Aaron Eagle happily attended Big Trees for three years, first all day as both preschool and day care center, and later as an after-school day care program when he started public kindergarten.

School is such a big part of a child's life, the choices made are crucial to the child's development. The stimulation Aaron Eagle receives at the hands of his teachers and aides in school are a major contribution for good or ill. If somebody doesn't like him for some reason, or has prejudice against his handicap, or can't control their impulses, then the child has to suffer this directly and without protection. We've run the gamut of experiences ourselves over the years, the best and the worst. By the time Aaron started public kindergarten, we had done the thing most often advised: buy a house in Berkeley. Berkeley has a reputation for being progressive, and it is in Berkeley that some of the best special education programs were started.

Aaron's kindergarten experience was a dream come true. He was assigned to a neighborhood school near our house, and we were told they would incorporate him into normal classes some part of each day. Our first successful battle with the school authorities was to get Aaron enrolled in the normal classroom every day, all day. Since he had been fully integrated at Big Trees for two years (he was the only special child there), we didn't see why he should be in a special education classroom at all. But the school wasn't accustomed to sending special children to class without an individual aide, and they didn't think it would be tolerated by any of the kindergarten teachers. We felt strongly that Aaron wouldn't need anything special, so we pushed for him to be able to attend on probation.

It was like a fairy tale. The teacher who consented to try having Aaron come to her classroom every day was the archetypal dream kindergarten teacher. Elsie was from Belgium, young and very open to the children, and she immediately liked Aaron Eagle and seemed to "get" him. She told me early in the year that they didn't normally test for social skills, or Aaron Eagle would have scored very high in comparison with many children his age. Aaron went to kindergarten every day and sat in circle with the other children, who learned to understand his language and reached out to nurture him in many loving ways. They befriended him naturally and came to his birthday party that year. The special education program worked effectively to support him and augment the work he did in the kindergarten class, such as making sure he was getting toilet training and speech therapy.

If kindergarten was a fairy tale, first grade (the first time through) was a nightmare. Aaron Eagle was no longer allowed to attend his classroom by himself but was required to have a full-time aide, and there were no aides available at the time. He began to cry every morning and refuse to go to school, and we didn't know why. One day I went with him to see how it was for him, and I was shocked to realize what was going on. In kindergarten the children had sat in circle and sang songs, played games, talked, and listened to stories that the teacher read from their picture books. Aaron had easily kept up and participated in ways that were fun and exciting for him. Now, in first grade, the children were sitting quietly at tables with pencil and paper watching the same teacher at the blackboard teaching them how to read and write. It was completely over Aaron's head. I felt very deeply for him, for the torture of not being able to understand.

The special education department had broken down over the course of the summer, with the director leaving and funding being cut. Things were unbelievably chaotic and dysfunctional in the special education classroom, with different aides coming and going every day, the temporary director sick or with her back out at least half the time, and a child with autism so upset that he screamed and hit himself much of the time, disturbing Aaron so much he never wanted to go into that room. If the teachers made him go in the room with the other boy, Aaron would become catatonic and go immediately to sleep with his hands over his eyes. It got to the point where Aaron Eagle wasn't even willing to walk into the special education room in the morning when we first went to school, he was so terrorized.

We put enormous pressure on the school, and then the district, in a vain effort to get our needs met. They said there were no aides available for Aaron, and none for the other boy, and they would have to attend the special education classroom. It was one of those perfectly miserable situations in which all the children suffered, and no solutions would work for everyone. The autistic child's disturbance was a clear indicator of the aura of trouble in the room, and Aaron's response to his screams (becoming catatonic) was also an uncharacteristic, but illuminating, way for him to behave. I kept bringing up the fact that if Aaron and the other little boy were as obviously upset as they were acting, then all the children must be feeling the tension and strain. I pushed for Aaron to be in first grade with a full-time aide, to no avail. With all the chaos and illness that seemed to sweep through the school that year, there was no resolving these issues. There were promises, always broken; time passing, another round of arguments, and finally (what a relief) the end of the year.

At the final IEP meeting that year, I sat quietly while the formalities were addressed so that the papers could be signed. Completely exhausted, I had it in my mind that we would get Aaron Eagle placed in another school before the end of the summer, so I wasn't paying attention to the details. Suddenly the speech therapist mentioned that she had given Aaron some standardized tests that the other children were taking, and she was surprised that he had not done well on them. She was thinking maybe she should not include the scores in his record! I almost blew up, I was so upset. I told her I couldn't believe they would spend the entire year not teaching Aaron anything, not even providing good custodial care for him, and then test him and wonder why he didn't do well! It seemed outrageous. I asked her to throw away the test scores.

It had been a hellish year for Aaron and for us, and then it ended, summer passed, and the school got a new director of special education. Everything changed under Barbara Trayler's influence—so much for the better, it is hard to imagine that the experience we have had this year is happening at the same place. Aaron Eagle is happy and runs to school every day. He likes being in the special education room part of each day, where he greets his friend, the boy who was so disturbed last year and who rarely screams now that he is surrounded by an aura of calm, patience, and individualized attention. We just erased last year and enrolled Aaron in first grade all over again, this time with full-time aides who accompany him all day. He is learning his letters and numbers and how to write his name. There is a well-adjusted feeling at school, as if everyone likes everyone else and is on the team.

Aaron Eagle is such a clown, he has taken to doing spontaneous imitations of everyone in the special education room where he spends a certain portion of each day. He can "do" all the kids with their characteristic gestures and voice changes, and then he adds lively renditions of the teachers as well. He performs this show for us regularly, laughing in good humor over his ability to capture the quirks and idiosyncrasies of each person whom he has come to love there. There is a level of stability and continuity at school this year that predisposes Aaron to success and a sense of self-esteem. Rose, an aide, takes him to class each morning and works on teaching him reading and working at the computer. Then after recess he does different activities with Toni, and after lunch Tia spends time with him until the end of the after-noon. Now and then there are substitutes, but not every day, the way it was during "the terrible year." He seems flex-ible and well balanced in response to the coherence and co-operative teamwork of the group of teachers, and they seem collectively interested in his well-being.

Last year there were simply no extracurricular activities at school. Every day was chaotic, yet predictable and bor-ing at the same time. This year, because of the healthy, easygoing manner of the director in the special education section, a flow of activities in Aaron Eagle's week includes swimming, cooking, and other fun things that the children enjoy doing together, as well as reading, making letters, and doing projects. They make music, work at a computer, and play outside, and Aaron Eagle has made personal friendships with some of the other kids with and without disabilities. He had a big party this year for his eighth birthday, with kids from school as well as other friends. People are relating to him, and he relates to others. It's very exciting to see the possibilities that open up to him in an environment where the prevailing attitude is that special kids are great and they can learn things.*

---

*In a bizarre recent turn of events, the school district suddenly—with-out explanation—terminated Barbara Trayler. Even though the parents of special children at La Conte School have protested Trayler's dis-missal, the district stands firm in its right to let her go. At this writing it appears that Aaron Eagle will have yet another unstable situation at school for no good reason. We are terribly disappointed.

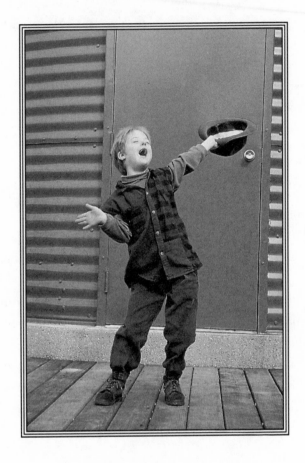

Aaron Eagle taking a bow, age eight.
Photo by Irene Young.

Chapter Nine

Whose Grief?

ڡ

B<small>Y THE TIME</small> I <small>MARRIED</small> J<small>ONATHAN</small> T<small>ENNEY</small>
and Aaron Eagle came into my womb, I had been a profes-
sional healer for many years. I used yoga and natural
methods of healing for myself and my children and meditation practices for my own spiritual grounding and self-
development. I had incorporated many of the Eastern
philosophies that accompany the practices of yoga and
meditation, but to these I added my own natural shamanistic tendencies. The earth-based, instinctual healing that is
practiced all over the world by tribal people has resonated
the most for me in my real experience.

The vocation of shamanism is obscured in the West by
layers of false understanding. I had naive expectations that

by being a healer, I would escape all the bad things in life and be rewarded in keeping with my ideas of goodness and perfection. I spent the first few years after my original spiritual awakening trying to perfect and purify myself as New Age esoteric texts recommend so that I would be "totally okay," that is to say, unafflicted by the things that other humans have to contend with. There is an implicit suggestion in New Age material that you can escape the "wheel," or the suffering that others must bear, by being pure, evolved, or "chosen."

I have come to understand that it's probably just the opposite. In our confusion, we've missed the point of spirituality altogether. To be "in service" means to carry more of the collective burden, not less! When a heart is open, awakened to the larger spiritual reality, then one sees beyond the immediate manifestations of illness and dis-ease into the hidden causes and cures. This is what it means to take on the task of healing, and the "call" carries with it the willingness to carry what cannot be borne by others. Shamans everywhere in the world live in community and not only share daily responsibilities like child rearing, cooking, farming, and cleaning, but also—in another role that is sanctified by their community—additionally act as spiritual counselors and wise women or wise men. Shamans don't get released from ordinary responsibilities because they are special. On the contrary, genuine healers add a collective burden to their personal existence in agreeing to be responsive to the needs of others.

Aaron Eagle didn't come into my life because I did
something wrong, failed to be pure enough, or needed to
learn hard lessons. He may have come because I offered
myself as a vessel for helping and healing. Certainly the
process of having him in my life has been a teaching, and
has humbled me, bringing me down to earth in a very direct and unavoidable way. Whatever fantasies Jonathan
and I had about our mutual task on earth, we have come to
understand what it means to be grounded in reality, vigilant and response-able every day. No airy-fairy task this,
but a deeply mundane and pragmatic necessity that presented itself to us through Aaron Eagle's arrival.

The nature of Aaron's condition made me feel needed in a
deep, almost desperate way. My own spiritual qualifications
for dealing with his condition made me feel good about taking the job. I felt that he not only needed a mother, he
specifically needed me, because of the way I tune into his
needs and respond to him in other than external, linear
ways. I see past his handicap to his soul. For many years, I
never felt what the experts discussed as the "chronic grief"
that I was expected to feel. I could occasionally feel something under the surface, like an inchoate complex of emotions ranging from being overwhelmed to wanting Aaron to
be "well." But it never really articulated itself into feelings of
wishing I didn't have him, or that he didn't have Down syndrome, or that I was being punished or hurt in some way.

Once I watched the movie *Gabby*, about a Mexican
woman with cerebral palsy who learned to write books on

a typewriter with her foot. The story was quite uplifting and amazing, but when it was over, I couldn't stop crying for an hour, and I didn't really know why I was having that reaction. I knew it had something to do with being Aaron's mom, but that was as close as I could get to a rational link with the movie itself. It had simply uncovered some of those nonrational feelings that go unnoticed under the surface the rest of the time. I am aware that this deeper strata of feelings exists, although I rarely encounter it so directly.

During Aaron's first six years, I went through my "midlife crisis," turned forty, created a career that included running a feminist school in Berkeley, publishing a quarterly journal on female shamanism, international travel, and publication of a new book. I produced community events, including the large one I described earlier where I first talked publicly about what it meant to be Aaron's mother. I did all this while maintaining my connection to Aaron and doing my best to be his (super)mom.

Then in 1990, my bubble burst. My school had to close; the magazine had to suspend publication, leaving me in debt; my marriage, which had been rocky for a number of years, finally collapsed. Grief-stricken, Jonathan and I managed to make our separation a healing one, in order to stay friends and devoted parents to Aaron. I felt alternately elated at my freedom and then exhausted and depressed. Now Aaron Eagle, like half the other kids in California, has two houses: Mommy's house and Daddy's house. When I travel, his dad is the single parent; when I'm home, I am a single mom. His transition was understandably difficult, and he was angry for about three months. But he has adapted in a healthy way, and although there is an emotional cost to his movement back and forth between two domiciles, the tension that he lived with when his parents were fighting has been eliminated, and he is clearly better for it.

I was fortunate enough to visit Bali in the spring of 1992. The people in Bali seemed free of conflict, living an ancient life of temple ceremonies and living off the land in extended families. Grown men carry small children, while women wearing colorful clothing walk with baskets of fruit and flowers on their heads. Their days consist of making offerings, watching over the rice paddies, solving community problems, attending and participating in dance and music performances. They seem at peace, and I've never been anywhere else in the world where there appeared to be no hostility between men and women. The place and the people made a deep impression on my psyche.

While I was there, I was able to visit a woman shaman of the older religious strata, the animistic and shamanistic layer that preceded the influx of Hinduism into Bali. This woman—called a Balian—lived in a village near where I was staying. A Brahmin man took me to her and translated for me. The format is simple: You go to where the Balian lives, with a question in your mind. You don't tell her the question. She goes to her altar in the private family temple, and, with her back to the petitioner, she begins to chant and pray to the deities. Then without ever having been told the question, she begins (in a deep trance state) to answer it quite directly. In my case, I was torn between two questions and was having trouble deciding which one I would "ask." I had an ache in my middle back, which had been causing the nerves in my left arm to go numb for several months, and I wondered if she could help me with it. But at the last minute, I decided to "ask" about Aaron Eagle instead, because I am always interested in what psychics and counselors have to say about him, and my curiosity got the better of me. As I sat in front of her altar, I held him in my mind, and she began to channel information from the ancestors in the ancient way.

I was shocked when the Balian began to chant and thump her back, right at the place where my pain and numbness was. Through the translator I learned that she was saying that my son was fine, he had chosen his life, and that I needed to "just love him" and not worry about him. She said several times that my husband and I should stop taking him to doctors. I couldn't figure it out at first, since we literally never take him to doctors! Then I realized she must be referring to the chiropractors we had been seeing. Two chiropractors in the Bay Area were working in special ways with Down syndrome, and we had started Aaron Eagle on a rather rigorous program of adjustments, which included a nasal adjustment that actually moved the bones around his pituitary gland. A doctor in Oregon (no longer living) had had many documented "successes" with patients who had Down syndrome; Jonathan and I had read about him, and one of the chiropractors we were seeing had been trained by this doctor. Although Aaron did not like the treatments, he seemed willing to have them, since he understood that we felt they were "good" for him.

What the Balian was saying to me touched me at a non-rational level. I didn't know why, but I cried and cried, and the place in my back that had been so tight began to release. I knew there wasn't anything wrong with what the chiropractic doctors were doing with Aaron. But she was telling me something different, deeper, about myself and my worried attempts to "fix" or change him. I realized we had spent the first seven years of his life trying to find the right solution, the perfect alternative healers, the miracle cure that would change Aaron Eagle's condition! In a book called *After the Tears*, Robin Simons discusses this tendency among parents of children born with handicaps.

> For some parents the insatiable need for "the best" masks another desire—the desire to "make up" to the child for bringing him into the world with a handicap. It's like saying, "We feel responsible for causing your problems, so we'll try to make it up to you by giving you the very best service we can find. (Maybe if we really give you the best, those services will cure your problems altogether.)"[1]

The Balian reminded me to simply love him, which I knew I already did, and she linked my lack of relaxation in relation to him with the pain in my back and the numbness in my arm. I would have never guessed myself that the two questions in my mind were in any way related. I didn't really understand it with my mind, but I accepted the information and let it begin to work inside me.

When I returned home from Bali, I had the worst case of jet lag I've ever experienced. After three weeks of being unable to participate in my life in a normal way, I realized it had to be more than the usual travel fatigue. Something about my visit to Bali had changed me, and I wasn't able to enter back into my life in the same way. I kept seeing in my mind's eye the green, terraced rice fields, the old temples, the natural caves in the rocks near the seaside. Everything here was going too fast—the traffic, the daily errands and routine comings and goings with their urgency, the constantly ringing phone with all the calls to be returned—and in the midst of it all was my own state of radical disengagement. I thought about moving to the country, being quiet, spending time in nature. I longed to be more calm with Aaron and to have less work on my mind and fewer tasks on my desk. But the structures in my life demanded a certain, almost impossibly vigilant focus, in order to pay my monthly mortgage and Aaron's child care and generally keep up with all the commitments I had already made to my work.

I had more trouble than usual relating to Aaron for the next three months. I felt deprived and overwhelmed with pressure, burdened with the labor-intensive needs and demands of my life with Aaron Eagle. The fact that he wasn't toilet-trained, and that it took so long to dress him, feed him, and do all the ordinary daily tasks of making his existence work, disturbed me, and I couldn't seem to get right with myself, or with him. I felt shocked at having these negative feelings toward him, and terribly guilty about it. The pressure built up inside me, and I thought I would burst. Meanwhile, I was teaching workshops and planning a month-long trip to Greece and Malta in the fall. The details were endless, the focus grueling. I was afraid I would get sick and ruin the whole trip.

Finally one day I got in touch with the source of my free-floating disturbance, and I began to cry. Like the original integration I had made in relation to Aaron's complex situation, here was another such movement toward wholeness I had to make now. I had to come to terms all over again with the realization that Aaron has Down syndrome, and it's possible that no matter how much I love him, no matter how perfect I am, and no matter what I do, I can't make up for it. Whatever language I use to free him, whatever terminology comes out of the disabilities movement, none of it takes away the extra chromosome he carries. The shaman woman's message haunted me: "Just love him." It seemed as if I might be finally having some of the feelings I was expected to have so many years earlier, when he was first born. I had a sense of why some parents feel hopeless at first and overcome with rage at finding out their child has a disability. And no doubt, as Robin Simons learned from the parents she interviewed,

The sadness, the pain, the anger don't go away. Even the most accepting, best adjusted, most positive people don't "get over" those feelings as they go on to make the best of their lives. The feelings are always there—under the surface—ready to be retriggered by new events. Birthdays, holidays, milestones (the year she would have learned to drive . . .), seeing other children his age, all tap into that well of "chronic sorrow."

The feelings don't go away—but they do get easier to deal with. Each time you experience them they are less intense. They are never as overwhelming as they were at the beginning.[2]

Something let go in me. I am growing in my ability to let Aaron be himself, without either pushing him to be something he is not or getting in the way of what he is. I feel as if some internal pressure let go behind my heart, and my arm is not numb anymore. There must have been a shadow hiding underneath my total acceptance and lack of emotion that, although it was unconscious, was having a psychosomatic effect on me. The acceptance that Jonathan and I felt toward Aaron Eagle and his particular condition when he was born came out of a sense of spiritual emergency. In that crisis, we handled things quite admirably, and our true and genuine feelings toward the entire situation were feelings of total acceptance and expectancy.

It is not the deep spiritual challenge that I find difficult, or the question "Why me?" that seems to haunt so many of the parents I've met, but the daily routines and monotony of life itself. Raising children is difficult enough, with the endless cleaning, cooking, washing, shopping, organizing, driving, caring, and paying attention that have to be done and redone hundreds and thousands of times for every child raised. Parenthood is a sacrificial occupation, one that insists that you step aside in many moments for the sake of this "other" that you have brought into the world. Raising a child with a disability is the same, but more so. The necessary focus on details consumes the creative hours of many days, and sometimes I just want Aaron Eagle to hurry.

Ultimately, even this daily, repetitive focus on the necessary tasks of the material plane—waking, dressing, feeding, washing, brushing, and always going somewhere—becomes a spiritual practice. Engaged Buddhism, it's called. Living life as if it were your meditation. Karma yoga. The patience that I must develop in order to greet each day with Aaron Eagle in a positive, life-affirming way brings with it the special qualities of compassion, understanding, and willingness. Simons quotes one of her parents: "Every day you overcome a barrier . . . then there's a new one." She continues, "The problems seem relentless. From frequent colds to medical crises, from skirmishes with bus aides to battles with principals, life with a handicapped child is not easy."[3]

What emerges in talking with other parents of children with disabilities, or in the insights that arise from my own experience, are descriptions of parents who feel they are becoming better people for the efforts they are forced to make. Words like *resilience* and *successes* show up frequently, as parents share the "storms they've weathered" and the "victories" they've celebrated. "You learn to take things as they come, not to look ahead and worry about what the next crisis will be. You just take every day, one day at a time."[4] This could be a statement from a twelve-step recovery meeting or a Buddhist teacher's lecture. The necessary courage, commitment, and carry through required make us feel stronger and more accomplished than if we didn't have this special child and the "extra work" he represents.

Aaron Eagle and I have been having a lot more fun lately, and we seem easier with each other as he grows. The admission, just to myself, that he is hurt ("brain-injured" as they say at the Institutes in Philadelphia) and it's not my fault, must have been a necessary one for my fuller and more integrated way of being with Aaron. Somehow I was overextending my own energy before in trying to protect against this and, in the process, hurting both myself and him.

Don't get me wrong. It's not that I expect less of Aaron now, or that he's not still my angel, my Buddha, and my teacher. He is all that and more. In fact, I'm beginning to see that I must let him take more responsibility for himself and stop doing the things for him that he can learn to do himself. (His special tutor, Alejandra, has been telling me this for years!) He needs the self-confidence of his own maturing, and I need to stop babying him. He is a person in his own right. My message to him needs to be less ambivalent, more certain: You can try it, Aaron Eagle, go ahead. My unfelt or unacknowledged guilt at being his mother (the one responsible for him) had made me hang onto him too tight, overcompensating, but my real love for him is allowing me to let him go. I am working now on letting him try and fail, and on knowing that I don't need to cover up his mistakes. I needn't bind him to me with unnecessary worry or ceaseless concern. I can be easier with him. He is who he is, and he is wonderful. And so am I.

Aaron Eagle is gentle and sensitive; he feels good about himself, but not at the expense of others. Like a monk, he is harmless. But he is hardly a sissy. He's got life in him, and I can hardly wait to see all the creative ways it manifests as he grows and develops into his full stature. His Self includes both male and female characteristics, and his ego is so simple that he doesn't know this is peculiar in relation to his particular culture.

I am reminded of what Will Roscoe called the Zuni man-woman, or *berdache*, the shaman role that has all but died out with European decimation of Native American tribes. A *berdache* was not a normal male or female, but not the opposite either. A shaman with very ancient roots, the *berdache* is pictured in rock art as androgynous, having characteristics and symbols that belong to both sexes. A Zuni *berdache* was someone who "occupied an 'alternative' gender," in Roscoe's research, a man who instead of being a hunter and warrior when he grew up, wore the clothes of a woman and did women's work. "The women of the family are inclined to look upon him with favor, since it means that he will remain a member of the household and do almost double the work of a woman" (because women take time out for childbearing).[5] He could move freely between men's and women's social worlds as a "nonwarrior or non-aggressive male, a crafts specialist rather than a primary producer, an individual who combined elements of male and female social, economic, and religious roles."[6]

Although in our modern culture we have no formal initiations as such, most of us attempt to demonstrate that we are one gender or the other. I grew up and married, had babies, and spent a few years in the traditional role of a woman. Yet, metaphorically at least, I believe I am a person more like Roscoe describes, being neither man nor woman in the traditional, sex-role-stereotyped way. Rather I'm a healer woman, androgynous, with a strong "male" spirit at work in me. Similarly Aaron's daddy has been described as a "feminine man." It makes sense to me that Aaron, with his unusual parents, might carry on this tradition and, in his own dignified but offbeat way, move back and forth between our two households. I so long for a return to ancient tribal ways, to when we lived in communities that worshiped nature together and didn't make war on one another, or on life itself. Once in Arizona I heard the red rocks sing, and since then I can't believe anything is inanimate or without intrinsic value. I dream of living close to nature with Aaron Eagle and other people, sharing life and work together without power struggles, without anger, in a world where we value the trees, animals, and everything on the planet as much as we value ourselves.

I took Aaron Eagle once to visit Camp Hill School in Pennsylvania, outside of Philadelphia. (It was a Camp Hill Village in Europe for adults where Nigel Hunt and his father went to live after his mother died.) Camp Hill is a community based on the principles of Rudolph Steiner where children with fairly severe disabilities live with others who are nondisabled, and they are able to function somewhat independently. The adults who live at this particular Camp Hill Village are "normal" but quite unusual, in that they choose to share life with special children whom they find beautiful and interesting. Households are composed of people with and without disabilities living alongside one another, sharing life, growing together, in ways that reminded me of a more ancient, pastoral time. The adults work there without pay, simply having their needs met by the community; they bring their children to live there as well. The commitment is strong; one of the men I spoke with had lived there for twenty years. Their stated view of people with handicaps is that one must relate to their souls, rather than their disabilities. This has always been my approach to Aaron Eagle.

Whatever grief I may yet carry in regard to Aaron's condition is more than balanced by the strange and mysterious paradoxes of his real life and mine and how well they blend. Aaron Eagle is a miracle to me, and watching him grow and flower is an open-ended journey that I am willing and eager to make with him. The ways in which he has softened his daddy and anchored him in the world are beautiful, and the ways he opens me and frees me from my limiting beliefs and patterns is an ongoing victory rather than a deficit. Aaron Eagle is a genuine healer, with a genetic and psychological legacy from his mom and dad, and he takes this tradition of healing proudly and seriously. Like shamans everywhere, he is an absolute original, unique and eccentric in the ways he brings relief to and takes compassionate leadership in his community. He responds to his call as well as any of us can. I am so very honored to know him, and I can't wait to see how his life turns out.

Notes

ॐ

Introduction

1. Thich Nhat Hanh, *Being Peace* (Berkeley, CA: Parallax Press, 1987).

2. Robert J. Mendelsohn, M.D., *Confessions of a Medical Heretic* (Chicago: Warner Books, 1980), p. 237.

3. *And Then Came John* is a heartwarming video on John McGowan's life as a child with Down syndrome, from growing up in Los Angeles to moving to Mendocino, where he was completely accepted and loved by the community. Telesis Productions International, P.O. Box 948, Mendocino, CA 95460 (707) 937-3048.

4. Jennifer Berezan, *Borderlines* (Chicago: Flying Fish Records, 1992).

Chapter One: A Magical Child Is Born

1. Cris Williamson, "Song of the Soul," from *The Changer and the Changed* (Oakland: Olivia Records, 1973).
2. *Kundalini:* In India, the word refers to the high-voltage energies awakened through yoga, or in this case through spontaneous experiences that generate healing energy in the body. *Kundalini* is said to be a giant snake coiled at the base of the spine, waiting to be awakened for spiritual enlightenment. When awakened, this Goddess becomes active in the body, rising through the spine to the head, bringing spiritual consciousness and awareness.
3. Thomas R. Verny, *The Secret Life of the Unborn Child* (New York: Summit Books, 1981).

Chapter Two: Instinctual Responses

1. Barry Neil Kaufman, *Son-Rise* (New York: Harper & Row, 1976); Nigel Hunt, *The World of Nigel Hunt: The Diary of a Mongoloid Youth* (Darwen Finlayson, 1967); Donna Williams, *Nobody Nowhere: The Extraordinary Autobiography of an Autistic* (New York: Times Books, 1992).
2. Glenn J. Doman, *What to Do About Your Brain-Injured Child* (Philadelphia: The Better Baby Press, 1990).
3. Patty McGill Smith, "You Are Not Alone: For Parents When They Learn That Their Child Has a Handicap." Information from the National Information Center for Handicapped Children and Youth, March 1984.
4. Felix F. De La Cruz and Joan Z. Muller, "Facts About Down Syndrome," in *Children Today* (Nov.-Dec. 1983), published by the U.S. Department of Health and Human Services, Office of Human Development Services, 200 Independence Avenue, Room 348-F, Washington, D.C. 20201.

Chapter Three: Energy Medicine

1. Dr. Henry Turkel, "A Superior Method of Treating Patients with Down's Syndrome or Other Storage Diseases," from *Nutritional Consultants*, September–October 1980.

2. "Help for Down Syndrome," from *East/West Journal*, December 1988. For more information, Dr. Turkel can be reached at 19145 W. Nine Mile Road, Southfield, MI 48075.

3. National Information Center for Handicapped Children and Youth, Fact Sheet Number 4, 1993.

4. Barbara Ehrenreich and Deirdre English, *Witches, Midwives, and Nurses: A History of Women Healers* (Old Westbury, NY: The Feminist Press, 1973).

5. Robert J. Mendelsohn, M.D., *How to Raise a Healthy Child in Spite of Your Doctor* (New York: Ballantine, 1987).

6. Robert J. Mendelsohn, M.D., *Confessions of a Medical Heretic* (Chicago: Warner Books, 1980), back of book.

7. Robert J. Mendelsohn, M.D., *Male Practice: How Doctors Manipulate Women* (Chicago: Contemporary Books Inc., 1981), p. 191.

8. Mendelsohn, *Male Practice*, pp. 192–93.

9. Mendelsohn, *Male Practice*, pp. 188–89.

Chapter Four: Wounded Healer

1. Robin Simons, *After the Tears* (San Diego: Harcourt Brace Jovanovich, 1987).

2. Barbara Tedlock, "The Clown's Way," from *Teachings from the American Earth: Indian Religion and Philosophy*, edited by Dennis Tedlock and Barbara Tedlock (New York: Liveright, 1975), p. 105.

3. Tedlock, "The Clown's Way," pp. 106, 108.

4. Tedlock, "The Clown's Way," p. 109.

5. Philip S. Rawson, *Tantra: the Indian Cult of Ecstasy* (New York: Avon Books, 1973).
6. Tedlock, "The Clown's Way," pp. 111, 113.
7. Joachim-Ernst Berendt, *Nada Brahma: The World Is Sound (Music and the Landscape of Consciousness)* (Rochester, VT: Destiny Books, 1987), pp. 117, 118, 119, 121.
8. Berendt, *Nada Brahma,* p. 112.
9. Sharon Burch, "The Chant," from *Yazzie Girl* (Phoenix, Canyon Records, 1989).

Chapter Six: Never Too Much Stimulation

1. Dr. Neil Harvey, Director of the Institutes for Human Potential in Philadelphia, private interview, March 25, 1993.
2. Glenn Doman, *What to Do About Your Brain-Injured Child* (Philadelphia: The Better Baby Press, 1990).
3. Doman, *What to Do,* pp. 222–23.
4. Doman, *What to Do,* p. 258.
5. Doman, *What to Do,* p. 183.
6. Doman, *What to Do,* p. 185.
7. Doman, *What to Do,* p. 193.
8. Doman, *What to Do,* p. 208.
9. Doman, *What to Do,* p. 209.

Chapter Seven: Trusting Psychic Perception

1. Arnold Mindell, *Dreambody* (Boston: Sigo Press, 1982), and *Working with the Dreambody* (Ontario, Canada: Arkana/ Penguin Group, 1989).
2. Brigette Hanf, "I Am a Hypothesis," p. 5. I am quoting from an unpublished paper about the psychic abilities of Hanf's autistic daughter, Eve. The paper was presented at a TREAT conference (Treatments and Research of Experienced Anomalous Trauma) in Santa Fe, NM, from March 17–21, 1993.

TREAT founder is Rima Laibow, M.D., a psychiatrist who worked with Eve. For more information, see Rima Laibow, "Dyadic Repair: A Clinical Approach to Autistic Recovery and Prodigy Retrieval," in the *Journal of ISSEM: International Society for the Study of Subtle Energies and Energy Medicine*, vol. 1, no. 2, 1990. To contact them, write to 356 Goldcoach Circle, Golden, CO 80401, or call (303) 278-2228.

3. Hanf paper, p. 11.
4. Hanf paper, p. 14.
5. Hanf paper, p. 13.
6. Glenn Doman, *What to Do About Your Brain-Injured Child* (Philadelphia: The Better Baby Press, 1990), p. 232.
7. Hanf paper, p. 24.

Chapter Eight: Mainstreaming Independence

1. Michele O'Keefe, "Count Me In! The Story of Jason Kingsley," from *Down Syndrome Today* (Fall 1992), vol. 1, no. 4, p. 21.
2. Nigel Hunt, *The World of Nigel Hunt: The Diary of a Mongoloid Youth* (Beaconsfield, England: Darwen Finlayson, 1967).
3. Hunt, *World of Nigel Hunt*, p. 22.
4. Hunt, *World of Nigel Hunt*, p. 29.
5. Hunt, *World of Nigel Hunt*, p. 30.
6. Hunt, *World of Nigel Hunt*, p. 31.
7. Hunt, *World of Nigel Hunt*, p. 38.
8. Hunt, *World of Nigel Hunt*, p. 40.
9. Penny Rosenwasser, *Visionary Voices* (San Francisco: Aunt Lute Books, 1992).

Chapter Nine: Whose Grief?

1. Robin Simons, *After the Tears* (San Diego: Harcourt Brace Jovanovich, 1987).
2. Simons, *After the Tears*, p. 72.

3. Simons, *After the Tears*, p. 15.

4. Simons, *After the Tears*, p. 16.

5. Will Roscoe, *The Zuni Man-Woman* (Albuquerque: Univ. of New Mexico Press, 1991), p. 22.

6. Roscoe, *The Zuni Man-Woman*, p. 145.